QUANTUM CHANGE

QUANTUM CHANGE

When Epiphanies and Sudden
Insights Transform Ordinary Lives

WILLIAM R. MILLER
JANET C'DE BACA

Afterword by Ernest Kurtz

The Guilford Press
New York   London

To Kathleen,
who lovingly changed my future
—WRM

To my son, Dirk,
whose arrival transformed my life
—JC

© 2001 The Guilford Press
A Division of Guilford Publications, Inc.
72 Spring Street, New York, NY 10012
www.guilford.com

Printed in the United States of America

This book is printed on acid-free paper.

Last digit is print number: 9   8   7   6   5   4   3   2

Library of Congress Cataloging-in-Publication Data

Miller, William R.
  Quantum change : when epiphanies and sudden insights transform
ordinary lives / by William R. Miller, Janet C'de Baca
    p. cm.
  Includes bibliographical references and index.
    ISBN 978-1-57230-667-7 (hardcover) — ISBN 978-1-57230-505-2 (pbk.)
    1. Change (Psychology) 2. Epiphanies. 3. Insight. I. C'de Baca,
Janet. II. Title.

BF637.C4 M55 2001
155—dc21   00-066340

CONTENTS

Part III. EPIPHANIES

Part IV. REFLECTIONS

ACKNOWLEDGMENTS

Our first and foremost gratitude is to the fascinating people who opened their hearts and gave us the privilege of hearing their stories of quantum change. The stories intimately convey, in firsthand accounts, the dramatic changes that occurred in these lives. They are powerful stories. One is changed in the process of reading them. Without the generosity and openness of these fifty-five individuals, there would be no story to tell.

We are also grateful to the interviewers who volunteered their time to hear and record these stories. Through skillful and patient listening, they called forth the rich detail found in this volume. All were involved in some way with the Department of Psychology at the University of New Mexico: Janet Brody, Nan Henderson, Mike Hillard, Dan Matthews, Henry Montgomery, Pauline Sawyers, Tracy Simpson, and Carolina Yahne.

Others were helpful to us in conceiving and planning the study. In Sydney, Australia, a group met regularly in 1989–1990 to think through how one might understand and measure quantum change; participants included Eva Congreve, Ken Curry, Loretta Elkins, Janet Greeley, Rian McMullin, Merida N'Enyar, Robyn Richmond, Steve Rollnick, and John Stanhope. Then in Albuquerque in 1991–1992 we were aided by preparatory discussions that included Lauren

Aubrey, Skip Daniel, Kathryn Grant, Jim Story, and Ann Waldorf. We are grateful to them all.

Finally, thanks to Ernest Kurtz, who wrote the Afterword, for his collegial guidance, eloquent scholarship, inspiration, and friendship over the years. We share his impassioned love of stories and of the deeper truths to which they point.

PREFACE

I have always been fascinated by the story of Ebenezer Scrooge. It has all the trappings of an engaging tale, of course: a masterful opening line; gradual revelation; ghosts, love, money, children, suspense; sharply defined characters; and the tension of good versus evil, of self-centeredness versus compassion. Yet beneath the narrative line there is something more that speaks deeply and directly to the soul and that accounts perhaps for the enduring appeal of this particular story. Like great mythology, it contains shadows of profound truth. Like monks copying and protecting manuscripts through dark ages, it preserves for us the ever-present human potential for remarkable change.

It was during a sabbatical year in Australia that I began to think seriously about how one might *study* such change. Rereading the Dickens tale, it occurred to me that I had seen sudden and dramatic changes happen in real life. Perhaps my daughter's own recent experience was the catalyst. I had seen Lillian shortly before we left for Sydney, and it was plain that something extraordinary had happened to her. I *knew*, I experienced in her a very different person from the raging teenager with whom I had spoken just a few days before. Sullen anger had been replaced with a peacefulness, with a gentle acceptance of what is and of what is not. I saw in her, at age fourteen, the sudden appearance of a quality I had not known in her before:

the capacity for genuine empathy, for seeing the world and herself through the eyes and feelings of others. There was a settled peacefulness and maturity beyond her years. It had happened, she told me, within the space of an hour. Unexpected, unbidden, and in the silent privacy of her own experience, something had changed her. She had trouble putting it into words, but at some deep inner level I recognized the experience. To be sure, the struggles of adolescence were far from over, but these qualities have never left her, and have continued to deepen in the ensuing ten years.

I remembered, too, a remarkable tape recording that was tucked away on a dusty shelf in my office, a letter from my friend Don. Our friendship began on the very day we met, and for three decades now we have felt a close bond. Even when we've not seen each other for a year or two, we can pick up as though we have been in constant touch. We simply understand each other without much explaining, as though living different versions of the same life. He had been driving across the desert, taping a letter to us, when an overpowering experience simply overtook him and literally drove him off the road. He turned the recorder back on and talked through the immediacy of it, and that experience became a part of this book.

There were others I had known over the years whose lives were changed suddenly, dramatically, and undeniably for the better. Much as I would like to say that these rapid turnabouts occurred in my therapy office, they never did. Some were profoundly spiritual and mystical in nature, one literally on a mountaintop in the former Soviet Union. Others were turnabouts without a spiritual or supernatural overlay. They are the dramatic moments of transformation that are the stuff of psychotherapists' dreams. Yet they seem to be of an entirely different quality from the usual, gradual changes that characterize people's lives, including their achievements in therapy. I began referring to them as "quantum change."

Scrooge, my daughter, Don in the desert, others I had met along the way—all mixed in my mind like old friends at a reunion, and the idea would not let me go: If such sudden, dramatic, and enduring changes do occur in real life and not just in fiction, I wanted to understand these transformations better, both as a psychologist–scientist and as a person who has always been curious about human nature and change.

I spent my early career studying how to bring about gradual, step-by-step changes and how to make them last. That led me to studies of what motivates human change, *why* it happens. Now I was faced with one of the most fascinating puzzles of all—the nature of quantum changes. How were they connected to everything else I'd studied? Why didn't they occur in my therapy office? Why did they happen to some people and not others? How enduring were their effects?

I began reading everything I could find and discovered that psychological science is pretty thin in this area. Instead, a picture began to emerge as I found pieces in fiction, biography, philosophy, theology, mathematics, and physics.

Still it was not theory but the real-life stories that seemed most compelling to me. Here were real people, not fictional characters, whose lives were changed forever in a matter of moments. Story, I sensed, is the heart of quantum change. Thus I set out, with the collaboration of Janet C'de Baca, to seek personal accounts from people who had experienced such changes. We had no idea what lay in store for us and just how many stories there would be. The ease of finding such individuals and the quality of their stories made it plain that quantum change is both real and not actually all that rare. We were struck by the diversity of the stories we heard, but also by some common threads that ran through them.

A year ago I would have said I had never had an extraordinary experience like Scrooge's—a sudden mystical encounter that transforms personality. I had had mystical experiences, but never one that triggered a personal metamorphosis. Since the idea of studying quantum change first took hold years ago, I have had the privilege of speaking to many people who have had such turning points, but until a year ago I would have said it was not an experience that I knew fully from the inside.

And yet it is. As we were completing the research for this book, we found that there seems to be more than one form of quantum change. Many who called us to share their experiences would preface their story with "I'm not sure this really qualifies, but . . . " and then would recount experiences that were clearly cut from the same cloth. Some were more like life-changing insights than mystical encounters, suggesting the two types that we have differentiated in this book. It was in this light that I made the connection to a powerful, sudden moment of consciousness that did set me on a new course, opening my heart to the adoption of our children (recounted in Chapter 4). It was, in many ways, the same phenomenon we had been studying through the stories of quantum changers.

What we learned from these stories is the basis of this book. In listening deeply to dozens of personal accounts, we began to see the commonalities. The stories have in turn caused us to struggle with the larger questions that led us to this project in the first place. What *is* quantum change? How do individuals undergo such rapid and dramatic transformation? The common tools and models of psychologists do not account well for such changes. From familiar principles of learning one would expect successive approximations, gradual small steps. To be sure, there are models of sudden insight learning, but these are usually focused on solving a particular problem. Are quantum changes the same kind of phenomenon, only larger? Could I, through scientific methods, come closer to understanding this phenomenon? These are some of the puzzles explored in this book.

One of the most intriguing questions to me is what happens in the years *after* a quantum change experience. I have mused now and then about writing fictional follow-ups to famous change-of-heart stories: What was happening five years after Scrooge met his spirits, or what ensued after the prodigal son moved back home? What is the rest of the story? In our research we gained a longitudinal perspective, talking with people who had, on average, more than a decade between them and their transforming moment, and thus we learned more about how these changes play out over time. But that is getting ahead of our story.

WILLIAM R. MILLER

PART I

THE CONTEXT

1

SOMETHING OLD, SOMETHING NEW

They appear to be in the nature of huge emotional displacements and rearrangements. Ideas, emotions, and attitudes which were once the guiding forces of the lives of these [people] are suddenly cast to one side, and a completely new set of conceptions and motives begin to dominate them.

—DR. WILLIAM SILKWORTH[1]

On the verge of losing everything that matters to him, a lone man leans over the bridge railing, staring down into the icy river far below. The business to which he has devoted his life is in financial ruin and will soon be controlled by his lifelong nemesis. He faces imprisonment, with the bleak prospect of leaving his wife and children to struggle for survival. The short plunge to his death would end his unbearable feelings of disgrace, and in an ironic twist the insurance death benefit would ease his family's financial suffering. Yet George Bailey will not die tonight. Something else, unexpected and implausible, is about to happen that will transform him.

In another wintertime and place, a solitary old man pauses in the doorway to his private quarters, escaping the chill of the street as he fumbles for his key. This day has been no different for him from

3

the ten thousand before it. Yet behind the door something uninvited and unwanted awaits him. This night will be unlike any other of his life, and before it is over Ebenezer Scrooge will be changed forever.

What accounts for the enduring appeal of these two very different fictional characters: George Bailey from the Frank Capra film *It's a Wonderful Life* and Scrooge from the Charles Dickens tale *A Christmas Carol*? Each is linked to the season of Christmas, just after winter solstice, when the darkest days of the year are past and there is just a glimmer of new light on the horizon. Their stories seem to rekindle hope in us, even hope against hope—the vision that new life is possible even and especially when it seems most impossible. Entrenched greed turns to generosity. Exuberant joy ignites from the ashes of ruin.

It would be easy enough to dismiss these stories as wishful thinking, a soothing balm to be applied at least once a year, as needed for relief from reality. They smack of the Hollywood happy ending. Sigmund Freud and Karl Marx would likely dismiss such tales much as they renounced religion as an immature fantasy that covers a darker truth. If these sorts of experiences merely occurred in fiction, no further understanding might be needed beyond an appreciation of their entertainment and palliative value.

The truth, however, is that such experiences do not occur only in fiction. They happen to real people, and not infrequently. They constitute a particular kind of experience with distinctive characteristics. Because contemporary psychology has no name (let alone explanation) for this phenomenon, we chose the term *quantum change* to describe it, drawing on both the concept of a quantum leap and the unpredictability inherent in quantum mechanics.

SOME HALLMARKS OF QUANTUM CHANGE

Even after ten years of listening to stories and studying quantum change, we find a precise definition elusive. Like spirituality, just when you think you've encircled it with a neat line, it escapes your boundaries. This much seems clear: *quantum change is a vivid, surprising, benevolent, and enduring personal transformation.* Each of these four elements seems to be important, at least subjectively, to the experience of quantum change, and we discuss them in greater detail in Chapter 2. Quantum change is *vivid* in the sense that there is an identifiable, distinctive, memorable experience during which the transformation occurred, or at least began. For Ebenezer Scrooge and George Bailey, it was one Christmas Eve when they were swept up by currents beyond their control. There is no doubt in the person's mind that something extraordinary has happened to them. An element of *surprise* is also clear. Quantum changes are not comprehensible as ordinary responses to life events. To be sure, external events can intervene in our lives as windfalls or tragedies to produce sudden, vivid and enduring personal changes. Though sympathetic, no one is surprised when a life is changed drastically by external events. It is only the intrusive events themselves that may be unexpected in such cases. Quantum changes are predominantly inner transformations, which often occur in the absence of any salient external event. A third striking element is the profoundly *benevolent* quality of the experience. To be sure, the immediate experience can be quite unsettling (as with Scrooge's ghosts or George Bailey's angel, Clarence), but there also tends to be an overwhelming sense of loving kindness behind it. Finally, quantum changes are *enduring*. They seem to be permanent transformations, a one-way door through which there is no going back.

WRITINGS ON QUANTUM CHANGE

Biography and autobiography offer many real-life accounts of quantum change events that were transformative turning points in the lives of people great and small. They are common among spiritual leaders: St. Paul and St. Augustine, Mohandas K. Gandhi (Mahatma Gandhi), the Buddha, Moses, St. Bernadette, Thesesa of Avila, Simone Weil, Martin Luther, Mary Baker Eddy, and John Wesley. They are found in the lives of social reformers and activists like Joan of Arc, Florence Nightingale, Malcolm X, Jane Addams, and Bill Wilson. They have shaped the lives of great writers and thinkers like Count Leo Tolstoy, C. S. Lewis, and Søren Kierkegaard.

Such events were well known and of great interest to William James, who is often credited as the founder of American psychology. In his century-old classic, *The Varieties of Religious Experience*,[2] he described a wide range of experiences and in particular discussed two different forms of change. By far the more common of the two is gradual, step-by-step movement, continual successive approximations as in the opening of a flower. Other changes, James observed, occur in a more sudden, discontinuous manner, and he speculated about types of people who might be prone to each of these kinds of change. Like Bill Wilson,[3] James was careful not to imply that one type of change is superior or preferable to the other. As a psychologist, he was simply interested in understanding how it is that people change so totally and abruptly:

> I was effectually cured of all inclination to that sin I was so strongly addicted to that I thought nothing but shooting me through the head could have cured me of it; and all desire and inclination to it was removed, as entirely as if I had been a suckling child; nor did the temptation return to this day.[4]

As we began researching quantum change, we were surprised to discover how few psychologists in the ensuing century had studied, described, or even voiced curiosity about this phenomenon. If it does indeed happen that people undergo pervasive and permanent changes in the course of a few hours or days, surely it is important to understand how this occurs. Yet, with a few exceptions, the response of psychology has been resounding silence. Journals and libraries are filled with knowledge about gradual change that occurs through learning and conditioning. Sudden discrete changes in circumscribed behavior, as through "aha" insight, have been described. Yet there has not even been a term in behavioral science to name this phenomenon of sudden broad transformation that is so widely described in art and biography.

Instead, the scholarly field in which quantum change has been described and studied most often is theology, historically an immediate ancestor of psychology. At the time of William James these were still closely related fields, making it only natural for him to study spiritual experience. It was later that a great chasm opened between them, with only the relatively isolated fields of pastoral counseling and the psychology of religion surviving to bear the family resemblance. It appears that the twenty-first century will witness some reconciliation of psychology and spirituality.

So it was particularly in the writings of theologians that we found good descriptions of this otherwise largely neglected phenomenon. One obviously related religious concept is *conversion*, which has been studied in some depth.[5] It is indeed the case that religious conversion experiences have some of the attributes described in this book, yet a common finding is that conversions often do not last. Furthermore, as will become apparent in later chapters, quantum changes frequently are not described in religious terms, nor do they usually lead to committed involvement in organized religion. Although they overlap, quantum change is a much larger phenomenon than religious conversion.

James E. Loder in *The Transforming Moment*[6] described a general pattern for experiences of this kind. They begin with the person being in a state of conflict and what Loder called "a rupture in the knowing context." Something disrupts the way in which the person has been perceiving reality and making sense out of life. This triggers the inner search for a new way of organizing reality, and sometimes in this circumstance "an insight, intuition, or vision appears on the border between the conscious and the unconscious, usually with convincing force." The experience is frequently accompanied by a great emotional release and a deep sense of relief. Then, with time, the person integrates and interprets the experience through language and symbols, and new patterns of thought and action emerge.

STUDYING QUANTUM CHANGE

To dismiss the phenomenon as fiction, one must believe at least that many biographies and autobiographies of great people have been doctored in retrospect with dramatic exaggeration of key transforming moments. Yet one also hears the stories in ordinary lives. It is difficult, in fact, to go through an entire lifetime without encountering at least one such real-life account. In twelve-step groups like Alcoholics Anonymous, such stories are downright commonplace. Once we opened to the concept and possibility of quantum change, in fact, we began to meet it everywhere. Whenever we spoke on the subject, there were people in the audience who had their own story to tell us.

So we began, in 1989, a process to study quantum change. At that time it remained an open question in our minds whether there was any observable phenomenon to understand. Perhaps, we thought, psychology had been silent on the subject for the good reason that there is nothing to explain. A decade later, that is no longer our question. The rich assemblage of stories represented in this volume has persuaded us that quantum changes are not only real but occur much more often than one might imagine. Instead, we are exploring the ramifications of a whole new set of fascinating questions about the nature of quantum change, its causes, and its meaning.

Perhaps one reason why this phenomenon is not more familiar is that people who have experienced such events are often reluctant to discuss them openly. Many who volunteered for our study voiced grateful relief to learn that there were others with similar experiences, often expressing a desire to meet them. Many had described their experience to only one or two others. Some told us that they had never revealed it to anyone else. Yet all were quite eager to tell us their story, and usually the words came tumbling out like a great unburdening.

Where does one find people who have had quantum changes? The answer turns out to be "almost anywhere," but we did not know that at the outset. We aroused the curiosity of a writer for the *Albuquerque Journal*, who wrote an engaging feature story with a sketchy description of quantum change in the widely circulated Sunday edition. People who had had such experiences and were willing to describe them in a confidential interview were invited to telephone our office. We had no idea whether we would receive any calls. We offered no payment for participation, and would be asking people to volunteer up to three hours of their time to complete interviews and questionnaires.

To our surprise, the telephone rang for weeks in response to this one article. Beyond many inquiries of general interest, we received eighty-nine calls from people volunteering to participate. A dozen declined when they learned the amount of time required or discovered that we were not paying participants. Another twenty-two later withdrew, were unavailable for interview, or scheduled one or more appointments but never appeared. In the end we completed fifty-five interviews, yielding a rich and moving array of personal accounts. These thirty-one women and twenty-four men were at many different points in the journey, with experiences as recent as one month and as distant as thirty-nine years ago. Most of them came from the Albuquerque area, though some drove a hundred miles or more to participate. As the ripples spread, we also began to receive letters and telephone calls from other states with still more stories.

We were invited to publish a brief report of our findings as a chapter in the American Psychological Association volume *Can Per-*

sonality Change?[7] It seemed a suitable place for our report, precisely because quantum changes often involve significant and seemingly permanent transformations of personality. Scrooge on Christmas morning was not merely behaving in some new ways—he was a different person, and that is the experience of many quantum changers. It's not that each of them became someone else, but rather that the same someone had been transformed. The transformation can be widespread, altering how the person behaves, feels, thinks, and experiences meaning. Our finished chapter provided statistical summaries from the questionnaires and interviews, and some observations about common characteristics of the participants' experiences.

THE REST OF THE STORY

It was clear to us, however, that the chapter did not adequately convey the essence of what we had learned and were learning. We had reported our data in scientific fashion, but we felt far from finished. In fact, we knew at another level that we had barely begun. We were personally captivated by the wonder and mystery of the stories themselves, and drawn by a still deeper story that we sensed within and beneath them. It was as if the scientist in us sat side by side at the campfire with a wide-eyed child entranced by a succession of master storytellers. Yet these stories were not make-believe but real, told by the people who lived them. Those stories became the heart and substance of this book.

Our aim is to tell you the stories in a way that captures the essence of quantum change, revealing some of the common elements and themes that we observed, but without removing the sense of wonder and mystery that remains with us still. The next two chapters round out a context to help you in encountering the stories. In Chapter 2 we summarize briefly what we learned by analyzing information that could be turned into statistics and describe in more detail some of the commonalities we found. This provides a high-altitude view of the forest, before we come to a more detailed description of the trees. Chapter 3 begins our walk into the forest. Here we describe what quantum changers told us their lives were like before their experience, and in particular what was happening just before it occurred.

The middle section of this book contains some of the stories themselves. It was difficult for us to decide, from over a thousand pages of transcription, which stories to include as illustrative. We have separated them into two types of quantum change that became evident as we studied them: insights and epiphanies (more on this in Chapter 2). The stories are told in the participants' original words, transcribed from our interviews. We have, however, removed all names and altered other potentially identifying details without changing the essence of each story. We did this to protect the story-tellers' anonymity and confidentiality, as we promised when they consented to participate and allowed us to convey their stories to you. Part II describes quantum changes of the insight type, and Part III recounts some epiphany stories.

The fourth and final section was by far the most challenging for us. Here we take yet another perspective by looking back at quantum change, first in the storytellers' own words, and then through our own reflections. We asked the storytellers what was different in their lives after their quantum change and how it had affected them. Their answers are drawn together in Chapter 16. We had anticipated that there would be just one final chapter in which we summed up our own understanding of what had happened, but then the questions grew and two more unexpected chapters emerged. The aftermath of quantum change seemed so consistently positive that we asked ourselves whether it is always so, or whether perhaps there is a shadow side, a darker form of quantum change. Our musings on this subject are found in Chapter 17. Next we do our best in Chapter 18 to make sense, as psychologists, of what it is that happened to these people, of what happens in quantum change. Perhaps you will reach different conclusions, but we have tried to relate commonalities in the stories to modern psychological theory and concepts. Still we were not finished. Something in the stories would not let us go. We close in Chapter 19 by drawing together some possible messages for humankind in general that seem to lie beneath the surface of these extraordinary experiences.

This is a map of the journey that lies ahead.

2

THE LANDSCAPE
OF QUANTUM CHANGE

The mathematics underlying three hundred years of
science, though powerful and successful, have
encouraged a one-sided view of change. These
mathematical principles are ideally suited to analyze—
because they were created to analyze—smooth,
continuous, quantitative change: the smoothly curving
paths of planets around the sun, the continuously
varying pressure of a gas as it is heated and cooled, the
quantitative increase of a hormone level in the
bloodstream. But there is another kind of change, too,
change that is less suited to mathematical analysis: the
abrupt bursting of a bubble, the discontinuous
transition from ice at its melting point to water at its
freezing point, the qualitative shift in our minds when
we "get" a pun or a play on words.
—ALEXANDER WOODCOCK AND MONTE DAVIS, *Catastrophe Theory*[8]

TWO TYPES OF CHANGE

Change happens. It is one of the few constants of life. Like a canoe
on a river, the question is not how to start to move but rather where
your current course of movement is taking you.

Usually change is gradual, cumulative, like drifting slowly down-

11

stream. Call it Type 1 change, or the "educational" variety, as William James termed it in his *The Varieties of Religious Experience*. You shift or drift a little bit at a time and, as with growing children, the changes may be most apparent to those who haven't seen you for a while.

Yet sometimes change also comes in big waves. Type 2 change is more like hitting the rapids. You are drifting along, and all of a sudden, before you know what has happened, you're moving fast and find yourself in a very different place. Every day some people's lives are thus changed forever in a matter of moments.

In many cases, Type 2 change results from the acts of humans toward one another or from the twists of fate sometimes referred to as acts of God. The results may be for good or for ill. In a popular early television series called *The Millionaire*, a mysterious and fabulously wealthy philanthropist chose ordinary people, not randomly but by some knowing and discerning process, to receive a gift of one million dollars tax-free. A cashier's check from the anonymous donor was delivered by a messenger, with absolutely no strings attached. The fascination in this dramatic series was what each new millionaire would do with the sudden and unearned gift and how it would change his or her life. The outcomes were sometimes uplifting, sometimes disastrous. Accidents, heart attacks, inheritances, storms, lotteries, fires, diagnoses, chance meetings, and bullets all permanently change lives each day. Sometimes it is a matter of just being in the right place at the right time or the wrong place at the wrong time. We try to insure ourselves against adverse intrusions and to place ourselves in the path of windfalls, but we remain subject to many external forces beyond our control.

CHARACTERISTICS OF QUANTUM CHANGE

Quantum change is a particular kind of Type 2 change. It may occur in conjunction with a significant external event, but in no sense can it be understood as a normal and ordinary consequence of such an event (at least not within current conceptions of change). It may be just as dramatic as natural responses to traumas or windfalls, but the drama tends to unfold within the person. People standing near an individual in the midst of a quantum change may have no inkling that anything important is happening. On the inside of that person, however, there is no doubt about it.

Vividness

It is absolutely clear to quantum changers that something out of the ordinary is occurring and that life will never be the same again. Through some identifiable, often dramatic, and usually quite memorable event, the person is transformed. It is utterly obvious to the individual that *something has happened*, something extraordinary.

Typically quantum changers can point to a particularly salient moment in which something happened to them. It may happen over the course of a few hours or days, but often it is a matter of minutes—"instantaneously," some say. The experience has a distinct beginning, though often a less marked ending, if it ends at all. There may be strongly ingrained sensory memories of the event: several people remembered a sense of brightness in everything around them; some remembered feeling cold or chills; others the feeling of incredible warmth. One woman found that "suddenly even the desert was pretty. I'm not trying to be poetic about it in any way. It was just like being given rose-colored glasses." Another described a specific feeling in her chest of "pain, suffocation, death" that was at the same time both agonizing and joyous. Yet another said that "the coffee tasted better. My vision had been widened considerably. I'm trying, but words . . . I have trouble here. It was sort of like instead of walking on the ground I was walking several inches above where I had been before."

A majority of quantum changers still recall the date, time, and vivid details of their experience many years later.

> *I just know that this experience made a difference in my life; it saved my life. It's one of the very few experiences that I truly remember, I mean in great detail, totally: everything I felt, everything around me, almost everything that was said and done, and the light. Everything. It's one of the few times I really remember.*

Of course, many people speak of how their lives have been greatly enhanced over time by things like sustained involvement in psychotherapy, twelve-step meetings, or religion. Their stories, too, are a testament to the human capacity for change. Yet such stories differ qualitatively from the accounts of quantum changers, who trace their transformation to a particular unforgettable experience.

Another form of vividness is that quantum changes are often accompanied by profound emotion. They do not have the subjective quality of reaching a rational decision or finding by personal effort the solution to a problem. They are often deeply moving. A very common experience during and after quantum change is a profound sense of peace and release from chronic negative emotions. There is frequently a sense of a great burden having been lifted. One woman, whose story is elaborated in Chapter 10, awoke one morning with the experience of being unable to initiate speech. For three days she had what she described as an out-of-body experience: "I could still see . . . myself. . . . I was kind of standing over on the side, and I couldn't talk. . . . [E]verything that came out of my mouth wasn't what was like me." Not surprisingly, this was quite an emotional experience, but she also found it soothing rather than frightening, "like when a mother holds a baby."

> *After that experience I just felt really peaceful and happy and glad to be alive, and every day since then it's just progressed more. The anger that was eating away inside me was gone. I've gained more confidence and I'm not afraid anymore, and I know what I can do with myself now. Whatever happens, I'm just at peace.*

Following his classic quantum change experience, Bill Wilson, cofounder of Alcoholics Anonymous, wrote this:

> *Slowly the ecstasy subsided. I lay on the bed, but now for a time I was in another world, a new world of consciousness. All about me and through me there was a wonderful feeling of Presence. A great peace stole over me and I thought, "No matter how wrong things seem to be, they are all right."*[9]

Surprise

Quantum changes are rarely remembered as willful or volitional events, like changing your mind or making a resolution. They are more like waking up one morning to suddenly discover that your skin is a different color.

More than four out of five people who told us their stories said that the experience took them completely by surprise. It was nothing they had expected, imagined, or even sought. It came unannounced and, as often as not, uninvited. If we had been able to ask them, on the day before it happened, whether they were in need of a personality overhaul, many quantum changers, like Scrooge, would probably have humbugged the idea. Many were not striving for or expecting a transformation. They didn't "do" it. It just happened. They had no map, and if they heard the rapids coming at all, it was only moments before they were swept up in the current. To this sense of unpreparedness and surprise, Abraham H. Maslow[10] added the observation that it also has the quality of newness, of having such an experience for the *first time*.

Benevolence

Almost always, the quantum changers we interviewed saw the experience as profoundly positive and beneficial, if not always pleasant. It is what Scrooge would likely have said, had we been able to interview him on December 26. The emotions experienced are quite positive, such as the intense joy and relief one woman in her forties felt when she saw a newspaper ad for Neurotics Anonymous and went to a meeting:

> *I was so happy. So . . . not just thrilled, so elated. I felt like I wanted to tell the whole world. I just wanted to burst into millions of pieces and go all over the world, and let a little piece drop on everybody and say, "Look what I've been given! Look at the joy, the wonder we can have in life!"*

To be sure, there are sometimes elements of sadness as well, perhaps of being sadder but wiser. A number of quantum changes told us they found that both joy and emotional pain were intensified for them. The contrasts were greater: "In many ways the experience intensified my pain also. Things seemed brighter and more beautiful. It was also a bleaker way of looking at things." Yet there was no question among the people we interviewed that the net effect was very positive. Sometimes there is a newly experienced sadness and compassion for the amount of suffering in the world, and a positive desire to take part in alleviating it. Less often in quantum change experiences there can be a new strong sense of responsibility and remorse for what one has done:

> *It was at that point that I began feeling extremely guilty about living with my boyfriend, who is now my husband. I didn't have that guilt before. I felt very ashamed of many things I had done in my*

past.—I started feeling the presence of what I interpreted as evil, where I had never felt that before.—I always thought that good and evil were just perceptions of an individual, that you created your own identity and your own reality.—I thought you could turn something that other people perceived as negative into something positive for yourself, and therefore there was no such thing as absolute evil.—But from that point, I have had a definite perception of evil versus good or whatever you want to call it, the Divine. I felt real sad from that point, and that lasted, maybe even to this point.—I just feel sad that I had wasted all that time and misled all those other people.—I wish I could go back and tell them.

Yet even such remorse tends to be accompanied by a sense of ultimate acceptance and forgiveness.

Many quantum changers voiced a deep sense of gratitude for what they had been given. When one hears of people who are "gifted," the first association may be of someone born with particular talents or aptitudes. The people we interviewed felt a different kind of giftedness. Each had received, in her or his own way, a unique and life-changing gift. Often it came as an unexpected flood of hope in a time of great darkness. Many voiced the clear sense of being in the presence of and gifted by a power beyond the self. The recipients typically felt they had no special qualities that made them deserve such a gift, but they were deeply grateful for it. Rather than opining that "I earned this," quantum changers are more likely to wonder, "Why me?" A woman who had been sexually abused by her father for years and who had experienced a deeply healing quantum change puzzled:

What I don't understand is why I came to all of this, to terms, to grips, when so many others who have been through the same thing as I have are not faring as well. They're devastated and broken and crushed. They have no hope. Nothing. They're broken, and they'll carry the scars forever. I don't understand why I've been saved or changed. Something's happened to me that they didn't get.

Another woman with a relatively recent experience told us:

When I heard the voice say, "You don't have to do that anymore; I will be with you always," I knew I could quit drinking. How can I tell anyone that I was able to stop that day and never have the de-

sire to drink again? Who would believe me? My mother is also an alcoholic and abuses prescription drugs, and she has been in numerous treatment centers over the years without success. I would love for her to have the same awakening that I have had. I wonder why this happened to me?

The stories of how quantum changers have dealt with their gift are quite varied. Some were embarrassed by the gift and sought to keep it secret even though some of its effects were clearly evident to those around them. Some puzzled long over what they were to do with it. Some simply accepted it graciously and rejoiced. Some felt a sense of responsibility, or at least a longing, to share with others what they had been given. Yet whatever they felt about it, almost all shared this sense of having been graciously gifted. "I was given something free," one person observed. "No strings attached. Ever had anybody do that to you, just give you something like that?"

Permanence

Besides vividness, surprise, and benevolence, quantum changers convey the sense of having passed through a one-way door. There is no going back. When you have just shot through a canyon in class five rapids, there is no way you are going to turn around and paddle back upstream. You are changed forever. Many of the people we interviewed in preparing this book still remembered the exact date and time when their experience began and had vivid recall of their surroundings and circumstances, even though the events had occurred, on average, eleven years earlier. It is plain to such people that they were markedly and permanently altered by the event. They were confident that what had happened would remain. Their understanding, their perception, had shifted markedly. Sea captain John Newton, author of the well-known hymn *Amazing Grace*, wrote of his experience, "I once was lost but now am found, was blind, but now I see." Having seen, quantum changers cannot go back to unknowing, nor would they care to.

When we asked people how their quantum change experience had ended, many said that it had not ended at all but was still continuing, still flowing. Their experience was not of a completed change but the opening of an evolution, a new capacity for seeing and understanding, a new link to the universe.

Vividness, surprise, benevolence, and *permanence*—together these words begin to describe the nature of quantum change. These are qualities that drew our attention precisely because these experiences are so different from the ways in which people ordinarily change. Normally, change happens a little at a time. It is hard to say exactly when someone became more wise or cynical, more intelligent or confident, more optimistic or selfish. Personal qualities wax and wane, one small step at a time, for better or worse. Having worked primarily with people who struggle with alcohol and other drug problems, both of us are well aware that change is rarely once and for all, a one-way door. This is one reason why quantum change is so fascinating and why the story of Scrooge has such enduring appeal. There is hope and capacity for change beyond our normal understanding.

TWO KINDS OF QUANTUM CHANGE

As we studied dozens of quantum change experiences over the years, they seemed to us to fall into two groups. The two kinds have much in common, including the attributes described above. Yet they also seem to differ in important ways.

The Insightful Type

Some quantum changes are best characterized as insights, such as one might imagine to occur in psychotherapy. Suddenly the person comes to a new realization, a new way of thinking or understanding. This new conception may pertain to certain life problems or circumstances, or to self-perceptions, or to life and reality more broadly. These quantum changes break upon the person's consciousness with particular clarity and forcefulness. The "aha" is deep and often of such magnitude as to leave the person stunned or breathless. From the moment of realization, the person is confident of its truth.

> *Toward the end of the time, a really great sense of peace and well-being enveloped me. And I knew—I mean I knew, not believed, not thought, I knew, as in one has truth or knowledge of— that I had made probably the most important step I would ever take in my life.*

Insightful quantum changes have a quality of growing out of life experiences. Although they occur in salient, identifiable, memorable moments, they tend to follow from the person's development rather than being an intrusion into it. There is a sense of continuity. When we asked people what is still the same, here are some of the answers they gave:

> My compassion for other people is still the same. I was a nurse before, and I'm still a nurse.

> I'm still hyper. I'm still real talkative. I still have some trouble with my temper. It's much better, though. That's something I've been praying, working on, getting some results with. I still like my home and my family.

> The physical world was the same; nothing seemed different. From that point on it just seemed like I had a different attitude. I had just had hope that maybe things would be OK.

> I'm totally different than I was. I am not the person I used to be, in any shape or form. Well, now, I take that back. Maybe there is one thing. I have strength. I've always been strong, a strong person. That strength has always been there.

Subjectively, insightful quantum changes are distinctly different from ordinary reasoning processes, from "coming to the conclusion that" or deciding. Yet they are not so far out of the range of normal experience. People may talk of these insights "as though" they had come to a conclusion or decision, yet the experience is distinctively different from ordinary conscious thinking and reasoning. There may be no immediate sense of being acted upon or in the grip of something beyond the self, as is usually the case with epiphanies, but the insights arrive suddenly, vividly, and with a sense of benevolent permanence. A man whose insight came as a dramatic and transforming surprise told us, "Instantly, I mean *instantly*, I saw things totally differently." Like several other quantum changers, he likened the instantaneous force to a lightning bolt. One woman described her curative insight as "an instant thought, a split second," and compared it to the sudden opening of floodgates: "It seems like it happened in a flash, and then that was it. There was no turning back."

The Mystical Type

Mystical transformations, or *epiphanies*, are experienced as quite out of the ordinary, qualitatively different from insightful turning points. In many respects they resemble classic descriptions of mystical experiences. Just as not all quantum changes are mystical, however, so not all mystical experiences lead to quantum changes. More commonly a mystical experience arrives, by invitation or surprise, and then passes on, leaving distinctive traces that fade within a few hours or days. It may fill the person with awe at the moment, but there is no sense of a turning point, of passing through a one-way door. The routine life that ensues is all too familiar. One man observed:

> *My procrastination hasn't changed. And I think, also, I take my family for granted a lot. In some ways that hasn't changed. I went through an incredible experience but still tend to dump on my wife and kids—to not treat her with the same sort of interest, conversation, or enthusiasm that I'd give to a stranger.*

With the mystical type of quantum change, however, the person knows immediately that something major has happened and that life will never be the same again. There is no question about it, and some would say there was even no choice about it.

It was tempting for us to say that the mystical type constitutes "real" quantum change. It is more dramatic, and in some ways a better and clearer example. The stories of Scrooge and of George Bailey are epiphanies. The stunning revelation of Saul/Paul on the road to Damascus is unambiguously out of the realm of ordinary experience. The insightful type of quantum change seems to have more continuity with ordinary reality (and for that reason, is easier to write off as "nothing but . . . "). Yet as we listened to personal accounts, we found that insightful quantum changes, while less startling and dramatic than the uninvited epiphany, seemed no less profound or lasting in its impact. As will become apparent, there are far too many similarities to arbitrarily designate one or the other type as definitive. Both tend to impart a mysterious and enduring sense of peacefulness. Both mark the beginning of lasting and often pervasive changes in the person's life. Both usually involve a significant alter-

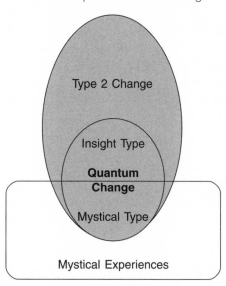

ation in how one perceives other people, the world, oneself, and the relationships among them.

What epitomizes the mystical type is the noetic sense of being acted upon by something outside and greater than oneself. Vivid recall for time, place, and details is more common with this type. Although sometimes coming at the invitation of prayer or a cry for help, mystical transformations are often unexpected and uninvited guests whose appearance, like Scrooge's spirits, can be most unsettling. Epiphanies also tend to be accompanied by the classic markers of mystical experiences more generally (such as temporary alteration of sensation and perception), which we will discuss in Chapter 10.

Are the Two Types Distinct?

Classifications of behavior and experience are always imperfect. Although we have distinguished two types of quantum change—the insightful and the mystical—there are experiences that seem to lie in the border region and are difficult to categorize. Many elements, as you will see in the stories, overlap both types, and their differences are small in comparison to their similarities. Our research thus far suggests that the two types are not completely separate but rather lie along what a statistician would call a bimodal distribution. The two types represent ends of a continuum. Cases seem to pile up at each end, but there are also some in the gray area in the middle.

The two types are meant to be a starting point. We found it useful and enlightening to describe quantum changes as occurring in at least these two common forms. There may be other types, or other classification systems may prove to be helpful. This is to say that one ought not to place too much importance on classifying every experience, or to be troubled if one falls in the middle and seems difficult to fit into our typology.

We have used the two kinds of quantum change as a way of organizing the middle section (Parts II and III) of this book. We will say more about each of the two types, conveying stories that show their similarities and differences. Before we look more closely at the insightful type, however, it is worth considering what was happening in the lives of the storytellers just before their experience occurred. It will give you some sense of the diversity of quantum changers before the change happened, the many starting points from which their lives began to converge.

3

BEFORE

Men's courses will foreshadow certain ends to which, if
persevered in, they must lead. But if the courses be
departed from, the ends will change. Say it is thus with
what you show me!
   —EBENEZER SCROOGE, to the Ghost of Christmas Yet to Come,
     in Charles Dickens, *A Christmas Carol*

Quantum change just seems to come out of the blue.
There is usually no apparent reason for its happening at that particular time, and like Scrooge, the person rarely sees it coming. For
about half of the people we interviewed, nothing special was happening at all and, until the experience began, the day had been no
different from thousands of others. One man was relaxing on the
beach during an island vacation, and another was just walking
through his kitchen. One woman was cleaning the toilet when it
happened, and another was sitting on it. They were driving, eating in
a fast-food restaurant, watching TV, walking in a park, working,
studying, waiting in a doctor's office, or sitting on the sofa at home.
They were leading ordinary lives as an attorney, a teacher, an Alcoholics Anonymous (AA) member, a physicist, a social worker, or a
single parent.

Others were in more unusual circumstances when it hit. One
was undergoing a backstreet abortion. Another was flying high on

drugs. One was on his knees in prayer for the first time in decades; another driving aimlessly in a strange city. A man embittered toward Christianity by virtue of his upbringing had gone to a monastery "in search of some peace and quiet" and found himself chanting with the monks. A woman who seldom attended church was driving to her parents' house after an Easter service. Another was at the end of her rope, at the bottom of desperation and on the verge of suicide.

Whether it began in ordinary or unusual circumstances, more than half of those who experienced a quantum change had been consciously unhappy, even desperately so. Some, like George Bailey, were transformed in the midst of a crisis or a dreadful tragedy: a man lying with his neck broken; a woman cradling a dying baby in her arms. Some were suffering chronic illness or great physical pain. Many said they had been unhappy for years or all their lives.

Then again, it's not all that simple to say who "needs" a quantum change. People who are leading peaceful, harmonious lives may seem unlikely candidates. For some like Scrooge, however, it was only in retrospect that they perceived they had been leading miserable lives.

Even for those who were clearly in misery, the question remains, "Why now?" Many had been suffering for a long time. Why did a quantum change happen at that particular time and not before or after?

HITTING BOTTOM

"I have met a number of people who have had experiences like mine," one participant observed. "The one thing that we had in common is that the experience happened from a point of desperation, where you don't know where else to turn. You come to the realization that you can't do it on your own, and you open yourself up to the possibility that there's something else there. As long as I was closed-minded to the possibility, I suffered in isolation. As soon as I allowed the possibility that there is more there than just physical reality, it happened. It was that immediate."

This reflects a perspective well known within AA—that one turns around (or is turned around) at the point of hitting bottom. Desperation was a frequent (though by no means universal) theme among our storytellers, particularly those who had had a mystical type of quantum change. Some had gone through a long period of suffering. One woman had just undressed for bed and turned out the light when she heard a voice that gave her a new sense of direction in her life. She described her prior life thus:

Even as a child I felt something was missing. I felt I didn't belong. I had friends, but I always felt like I was not in touch with reality, that I just really didn't belong. I went through two marriages and felt like I was a complete failure. I was always searching, never satisfied. I was trying to pull myself together from the second divorce. I dreaded getting up in the morning, just hated the thought of having to face another new day. I felt completely worthless, like I had been an absolute failure. I had been searching desperately. I cried all the time. I knew there had to be something else. I knew that I needed something.

For another, the long and painful deterioration of her family led up to a quantum change:

My daughter was breaking up her marriage. I thought my son was going crazy, and my husband was drinking. My whole world was falling apart, and I felt that I had nothing to hold on to. I used to look out my window at the neighborhood and think, "There are all these people out there, and nobody knows what we're going through." My husband couldn't help me because he was just devastated, and the only answer he could think of was to have another martini. Because of my husband's prominent position, I couldn't talk to people about what was happening. I wasn't even telling my mother much about this.

One night after our son had gone to bed and my husband was gone, I remembered there was a gun in the house. It was a forty-five, a big gun. I thought, "Life is not worth it, and I can't go on this way." I thought I could shoot my son—I'd have to take him with me—and then shoot myself. It was not an idle thought. I thought, "This is the way out, there's no other answer." I went to bed, and I couldn't sleep. I just tossed and tossed all night long and said, "What am I going to do? What am I going to do?" I felt total despair. I just had reached rock bottom. I couldn't go down any further.

It was at this moment that it happened. "Suddenly it was

like this angel appeared in my mind and said, 'Turn to me.' And that was it—just like that. It wasn't from anybody else, or like I saw a blinding flash or anything. I just turned to the divine and knew that everything was going to be all right."

Another mother, whose story is continued in Chapter 10, had reached the end of her rope with a rebellious daughter when she had a quantum change that brought her "a wave of assurance":

It was in the middle of the night, a Friday night. My husband was out of town. He was usually gone on Friday nights, and this is when most of the acting up took place. This particular night she came in and went to bed. I had waited up for her, or maybe I woke up when she came in—I don't remember which. Then I awoke again a little later, and I went and checked her room, and she was gone again. I remember going back in the bedroom and just falling on the bed and beginning to cry. Very emotional. I had plopped on the bed face down. I thought, "I've done everything I know how to do. I just can't do anything else." I was so disturbed to find out for certain that she wasn't in her room and that she had lied to me again. I was crying. I was desperate. I really didn't know what else I was going to do. I had tried everything. I had even threatened to chain her to the kitchen sink at one point, which made us both laugh, but I just felt so helpless. I just didn't know what else to do. I said, "Oh dear God, help me. What can I do here? You're going to have to help me. I just can't handle this."

TRAUMATIC CHILDHOOD

Another frequent theme was of traumatic childhoods. Often these individuals had developed victim identities, and not without reason. Some had been abandoned. One teenager woke up to discover the bodies of both parents after a murder-suicide. Several women and men had suffered severe abuse for many years. One woman recounted this story:

Starting when I was five years old, I was sexually abused by my father. As I grew up, I tried to get out of the situation. I went to my mother, and she didn't believe me. I couldn't go to the police, be-

cause my father was the police and he had a lot of power. Who would believe a little girl? Back in those years, that kind of stuff wasn't out of the closet and you didn't talk about it. In fact, my father threatened to send me away if I didn't keep quiet. He would've too. God knows where he would have sent me. So I suffered right through my teenage years. I was basically turning into the biggest drunk and harlot that you ever did see. I ran away and got married to try to get away from my father and his men, but he still kept bothering me. He was still stalking me when I was twenty-five. My marriage, of course, went down the drain. I just felt I was never going to get out. I was sinking, and I felt that I would die there. After a while I stopped trying to get out and just spent my life in bars with other men. I would have killed myself eventually. I entertained the thought several times, to get out of the mess. I had no real love for anyone or anything. I saw no reason for my existence. I wasn't contributing to anything. I wasn't going anywhere. I just spent my time in bars and having fun, or what I thought was fun.

Her transforming moment came "out of a clear blue sky" when something inside told her to move to New Mexico. "It was just like bells and goosebumps," a clear knowledge that this was the right path for her. "I straightened out. I don't drink. I don't do drugs. I have a beautiful family, and I've made a life for myself."

TRAPPED

The sense of being trapped, of having no way out, was evident in a number of stories. All of the possibilities had been used up. All routes of escape had been blocked. Everything had been tried, and there was no hope. One woman in her thirties was living with her parents:

My parents are very thumbs-on people. I had no real personal freedom. I was caught in this trap, and I couldn't do anything. Even though I was thinking for myself, I couldn't release myself from the situation I was in. My dad was always putting me down, being very negative and rude, and my mom was a very weak individual and never stood up for me or herself. I wasn't depressed, but I just couldn't do anything. There was nothing that was important for me in life. I knew that I would never be able to get a job and be happy. I knew I would never have a family because I was past my twenties, and I still couldn't succeed at the university because every time success was close I'd just freeze up and fail on purpose. So there just was no way I was going anywhere. My life was terrible, and it was just emptiness. There was nothing there.

One day she was watching TV, alone at home in her mother's house, when she suddenly realized that something unusual was happening:

It was a kind of pull. I can still see in my mind. It was like there were some people who were saying "Come with us for a minute," only they really weren't saying that. They were just more or less beckoning. My first response was "No way." [She laughs.] That didn't seem to stop it, though. My own will was sort of moved over to the side and I could still see me; I could see me here and I could see me there. It was like there were two of me, 'cause I could see both things.

Another woman had grown up extremely fearful, with dire warnings from her parents throughout childhood of the many terrible things that could befall her in the world. On the night her quantum change happened, she was babysitting on New Year's Eve and became terrified because unbeknown to her the family had moved and she didn't know where she was:

So there I was in a strange house, I didn't even know what street I was on, and it was already dark. It was like a trapped situation, and I started searching frantically for envelopes with an address on them so I could know where I was to call the police. Every sound— the wind, a dog scratching at the door to get in—everything frightened me. I worked myself up into it like adolescents can do, until finally I was standing in the middle of the room just turning and turning to make sure nobody was coming up behind me.

AIMLESS WANDERING

Another theme that emerges with some frequency as a precursor to quantum change is a sense of wandering aimlessly. One might infer a search from such wandering in the wilderness, but the person's own experience was one of purposelessness, just drifting from day to day. Some were lost in a haze of alcohol and other drugs. Some lives had been passing from day to day in mindless routine, moving through years with a vacant stare. Perhaps they were running *from* something, but there was no sense of moving *toward* anything. The days just passed. Before the quantum change struck them, they had not been consciously looking for deliverance from their stagnation.

RELIGION AND PRAYER

We asked people about their religious backgrounds, because we were curious about how it might affect quantum change. At the very least, one's religious background may influence the way in which one understands and interprets such experiences. Before and after quantum changes, a broad spectrum of religious belief was represented: Catholic and Protestant, Islamic and Jewish, Buddhist and humanist, agnostic and atheist. While many of the features of quantum changes were similar, the meaning and interpretation given to them varied widely, guided in part by the person's prior conceptual framework. Some who had mystical experiences, for example, interpreted them as being touched by or in the presence of God; others experienced a more Buddhist-like oneness with the universe; or experienced awe without an object. There were some conversions from one religion to another, and to a new religion from none. In short, the religious context of quantum change experiences varied widely, and for some there were no spiritual or religious overtones at all.

What did strike us as frequent in the background of quantum changers, however, was a report of alienation from a religious tradition that the person had once experienced, whatever it was. A woman whose quantum change moved her from atheism to being "deeply spiritual but not religious" said of her earlier life:

> *I was so glad to get away from religion. My mother insisted I go to church, and that was an important part of my life that I rebelled against. I enjoyed breaking all the rules of the church, and when I married I decided to drop the whole thing. I wasn't going to have anything to do with religion whatsoever, and I devoted myself to having a good time.*

For others, the alienation had been through disinterest more than re-jection:

> *I had a spiritual life before this, a faith in God, but I would use it*
> *only in crisis. My parents were not religious. My dad's an atheist,*
> *but they sent me to Presbyterian Sunday school to just get a basic*
> *understanding of Christianity. Then I drifted into being Unitarian*
> *for a couple of years, and then completely out of formal religion for*
> *probably ten years. About five years ago I rejoined the church and*
> *was baptized as a Christian. But my spirituality as an adult was*
> *still pretty watered down. It was there, but it was nothing compared*
> *to what I feel now.*

Often, however, there had been not detachment or disinterest, but lingering anger and bitterness about religious upbringing:

> *I was raised in a Catholic home and attended a Jesuit school. I had*
> *many questions about the world I lived in and about God. By the*
> *time I was in high school, I considered myself an agnostic. As I got*
> *older I was probably more of an atheist, even to the point where I*
> *was aggressively antireligious. When I saw people who were reli-*
> *gious, I thought maybe they were using it as an escape and hadn't*
> *thought seriously about their lives or the world around them.*

Others harbored resentment about guilt imposed by religion:

> *I had gone to a church where all these sins and guilts were laid on*
> *you. I was told that if you're divorced and then marry again, you*
> *commit adultery.*

Nevertheless, the seeds of religion sometimes gave the person somewhere to turn at the bottom, when all other hope had been ex-hausted. About one-third of our quantum changers were praying when it happened, sometimes the first prayer they had offered in many years or ever. Prayer was, in fact, the single most common act preceding quantum change. It was in this context that some quite in-tense mystical quantum changes occurred:

> *One night I was walking about in Harlem. I enjoyed the people*
> *there, and I was fine. Nothing untoward ever happened to me in the*

*streets there. In fact, I kind of like the street life in New York. But
my life had begun to turn sour because of drinking, carousing, infidelities. The whole pace of that life was nuts, and the man I was
living with was also not well balanced. There was abuse, physical
abuse of me, and lots of infidelities, which created a real violent
home life. The whole situation just began to disintegrate over a period a time. So anyway, I was tootling up to the club to hear some
famous jazz group and to meet my man, and on the way I saw an
incident happen in the street with a man and a woman who I think
were tipsy. They weren't real real drunk, but they had an argument
and he hit her and her purse went flying. It just shook me up. That
kind of thing does that to me. I kept walking and thinking, "Hey,
this is not where you want to be." I got more and more depressed,
and I made the first prayer I had made in many, many years. I was
raised a Roman Catholic, in a time when it was very, very Catholic—you know, in the forties and fifties, taught by the nuns at
school, and living in an orthodox Catholic home. I had left all that
behind when I went to college. I dropped out of college to become a
beatnik. So I made my first prayer in years and years, and I said a
very simple thing. I said, "God if you exist, get me out of this, cause
I can't do it by myself. I am a lost woman here."*

As she prayed on her way to the nightclub, she passed a newsstand
where she saw and purchased a paperback copy of Thomas Merton's
autobiography, *The Seven Story Mountain*. She turned around and
went home: "I stayed up all night reading it. I was in tears when I
finished the book. It just turned me around. The next day I bought a
Catholic medal to wear. I started praying. Here I am living in Harlem
with my boyfriend, planning how I might become a monastic nun."
Ultimately she became a civil rights activist and a social reformer.

Another was an addicted physician who had been stealing and
injecting opiates. Despite the obvious threat to his license and career, he found himself unable to stay away from drugs:

*I got real suicidal and was thinking of killing myself. My elaborate
suicide fantasy was that I would go into the morgue, inject KCl,
and I would then swallow my suicide note so that when they did
my autopsy, they would cut open my stomach and find the suicide
note. Aren't I creative? But I realized I couldn't do this suicide thing
to my beautiful children.*

When he was in college, he had decided, "Who needs God if you're going to be a doctor?" Now, in the depth of desperation, he tried for the first time in his life what he had been told to do in AA meetings:

> *My first prayer was something like "God, I don't know if I believe in you really. I don't know if you're there. But I do know I'm miserable. Please help me."*

There followed a mystical experience, recounted in Chapter 10, through which he was freed of his drug addiction.

All of these factors are frequent in the background of quantum changers. Yet the phenomenon refuses to be so easily pinned down. There are exceptions to every rule. There were those who could point to nothing at all out of the ordinary that preceded their dramatic change. If we had to describe in a few words the most common candidates for quantum change, they would be people who were desperately unhappy, had been for some time, and saw no way out through their own willful efforts. Yet even this broad generalization characterizes only about half of those who told us the stories that follow. For better or worse, many others were mostly living their ordinary lives.

Then it happened.

PART II

INSIGHTS

4

THE INSIGHTFUL TYPE
OF QUANTUM CHANGE

When the answer begins to come, it does so in a
startling way. . . . You will either see it or hear it, and
you are often given a great deal of knowledge in a brief
period of time. It is a powerful experience that almost
overwhelms you.

—FOOLS CROW[11]

ANATOMY OF AN INSIGHT

On the Island

*My wife and I were away on an island vacation, and it was mid-
afternoon. I remember the sunlight on the water, and all the green;
that's still fixed in my mind. My wife was out on the water, and I
was relaxing and doing some reading. I had been worried about one
of our employees, whom I viewed as having some alcohol-related
problems. I had learned from him that he was the adult child of an
alcoholic. Both his mother and father were alcoholics. I was trying
to learn some more about that, so that I could work with him better.
I had taken along a couple of books. They were talking a lot about
codependency and the behavior patterns of adult children of alcoholics, and I began in that process to see some things in myself that*

I was really unhappy with. I didn't like the way I felt after a good night of drinking. I'd get up the next morning with a foggy head and just not feel particularly good. I was unhappy with some weight that I was carrying. I was heavier than I wanted to be from all the calories in the alcohol, though I didn't realize it at the time.

Now, I had been a real avid runner and exerciser, an aerobic exercise buff, but I had let the pressures of my job become a reason not to find time for the exercise. So I decided, while my wife was out on the water each day, that I would do something for myself, get out and walk on the island. I started taking long afternoon walks down these deserted roads out there, reflecting on some things. I did a little bit of running and I found, God, I couldn't even run a quarter mile. At one point I had been up to marathon trim.

I guess it was that, and some things that were coming out of the reading I had taken along to try and get a handle on how to help the employee. I decided, "I have a problem with alcohol, and the only way to deal with it is to simply put it aside." And all of a sudden, it just dropped away. At that moment I turned into somebody who didn't use alcohol. I haven't had a drink since that day two years ago. I can't even remember the last time I had a drink.

Three nights later, we went out to dinner with some people my wife had met. I thought to myself, "I'm not going to have a cocktail. I'm going to do something different. I'm going to." I remember drinking a club soda with a twist. Now, I hadn't shared this with my wife yet; I didn't tell her that I had stopped. This was an internal decision. I didn't share it. I was just talking to myself. I remember the surprise on her face: "Aren't you going to have something to drink?" I said, "No, I don't think I will." I didn't and haven't, and that was that. I knew for sure at that point that something was happening inside, because that was not the old me.

"I Just Decided"

For years we have been interested in how it is that people make significant changes in their lives. Most people who quit smoking or drinking do so without seeking professional help. At any given time, about one in every ten or eleven adults in the United States have significant life or health problems related to their own use of alcohol. Long-term follow-up research shows that most of them get through it. Find them five or six years later, and most of them are no longer drinking in a way that causes problems. By any stretch of the imagination, only a fraction of them could have received treatment or even mutual help such as AA.

How did they do it? Perhaps if we understood what happens in such natural change events, we could find better ways to help people who want to change.[12] Yet, when one asks such people how they did it, they often have a hard time being specific and tend to say something like "I just decided." It's what the man whose story opened up this chapter might say if you asked him casually how he stopped drinking.

Sometimes it *is* a simple decision, a logical, willful process. People weigh up the pros and cons and come to the rational conclusion that change is needed. That sets the process of change in motion. They may or may not succeed on the first try; and often they don't. Nevertheless over time they reach their goal. It can be a Type 2 change, sometimes sudden, but not what we mean by a quantum change. It lacks the usual subjective elements of vividness, surprise, passion, and a sense of giftedness.

Buried in the statement "I just decided," however, can be another kind of experience that has been confused with ordinary decision making. It is the insightful type of quantum change. When people talk about such experiences in shorthand, they may say "It just happened" or "I just decided." Inquire a little more closely, however, and it becomes apparent that the process is somewhat more complex. It is tempting to use shorthand, because like all quantum changes, they can be difficult to explain in words. In the language of the gentleman whose story is given above:

> I'm not sure if you can describe it in words. I'm struggling with that one. It's very . . . I can't quite say what was going on. I wish I could. It would be fun to speculate, to try. I can't describe the process, and I can't quite precisely put my finger on what was going on. It was not a flash of light or a burning bush or anything like that, but there was definitely something happening inside. I can't quite describe it. I can't quite articulate what some of the feelings were.

Sometimes people find it helpful to talk about what happened through metaphor:

> I wouldn't say it was a flash of revelation, but it was sort of a cumulative set of insights. Maybe, maybe it's the way a crystal forms. You can watch it sort of come together, and then as all the pieces are in place, it solidifies. It's hard to say exactly when it stops being liquid and becomes crystal, but there's a point at which it changes property. I felt a change of property.

Looking back at the experience, people also struggle to assimilate it within their larger frame of knowledge and beliefs. Reflecting on the foregoing island experience, the man added:

> I am a spiritual person. I'm not hooked into any kind of organized religion, to doctrine and stuff, but I have a high level of belief in things that are spiritual. I suspect that this was a spiritual insight of some kind, that it was given to me. Whether I was allowed to have it, I don't know the mechanisms. I'm not sure what it was about, but I ascribe it to a power outside of myself, a power higher than myself, a power beyond myself. Maybe I was at that one moment ready to listen. Maybe a whole set of things converged so that I could suddenly hear what was being offered.

Insight as More Than Cognitive

This man did more than stop drinking. His identity suddenly changed from that of a drinker to a nondrinker, which proved to be particularly illustrative in another way. Years earlier he had quit smoking, and the two experiences were quite different to him subjectively. He talked about the difference in this way:

> I used tobacco for many years. I used to smoke cigarettes, and it was interfering with my lung capacity and my running, so I quit. This is twenty years ago, I quit. I found one of those four-week programs, and I went through it. By the end I had weaned myself off nicotine and realized how hard it was, and I decided that I didn't want to go through the hard part of weaning myself off again. But it was not at all the same. There was no comparison. It wasn't a

self-awareness where I changed the paradigm or changed my head and said, "I am not a smoker. I don't use tobacco." That's what happened to me during that walk on the island. That certainly wasn't what happened with tobacco. I mean, it was such a pain in the butt to give up the nicotine that I said, "That's too much work. I'll never do this again." It's a very different kind of change. That was a change, too, but it wasn't a growth change as much as this was. How do I describe the difference? What I've gone through to me is growth. With the tobacco, I simply broke a bad habit. For me, alcohol wasn't a habit. It was a feature of me. Now, there's the difference, right there. The nicotine was a habit, an addiction. The alcohol was a feature of my being. I had to reconfigure myself, or something helped me reconfigure myself.

It is difficult to find a good word for that sort of experience. We have chosen *insight* as a concept that encompasses this kind of crystallization, at least as the term has been used historically within the field of psychotherapy to refer to a kind of breakthrough realization. Beware, however, the popular connotation that insight is a purely cognitive phenomenon, a dispassionate or logical conclusion. This quantum kind of insight involves the whole person—thoughts, actions, emotions, and spirit—and in some ways represents a change in the personal sense of self. Like quantum changes more generally, it happens within a relatively brief period of time and breaks upon consciousness like a forceful wave. It is compelling and often accompanied by substantial emotion. This is one reason that such experiences are so memorable. Again, reflecting on the same island experience, the man noted:

It's as with any other thing that is emotionally powerful—where you were when you heard the news about Kennedy's assassination, or where you were when you heard about the launching of the first strikes in the Gulf War—anything emotional. It lays down those long-term memory traces quite effectively, and they're there to really recall. At the time I didn't realize it, but I can recall vividly the light patterns, texture, the context of some of that walk in a quite clear way. It is clearer to me now than I would at the time have thought I'd be able to remember it. I can remember where I was, what I was doing, what some of those thoughts were of, well, "It's your problem." They come back to me. Some of it is talking to my-self, I guess, but there's some emotion, too. There were some emo-tional things that happened, and that is how I can remember this so clearly.

All of that can lie beneath the deceptively simple explanation, "I just decided."

INSIGHTFUL CHANGE

Small insights are the "aha" experiences of everyday life: realizing what someone means, seeing the solution to a puzzle, getting the punch line of a joke. To apprehend something that one did not per-ceive a moment before is a common process.

Quantum change insights also involve a shift in perception and the realization of a new reality, but at a much deeper level. "I don't drink" was not experienced as a willful decision but as the sudden realization of a new identity: "I am a person who does not drink." It is as though a new pair of glasses suddenly brings the world into clear focus and, having seen, the person can no longer envision it as before. "I was blind, but now I see" is one image. Another is the shift from seeing the world as a child does to understanding it with an adult mind.

Not only is there a sudden new perception, but the person in-stantly recognizes it as authentic truth. This is often accompanied by an immediate awareness that something permanent has happened— a transformation has occurred:

Right then, I knew that I would never be the same.

I just knew that I would never have another drink.

Something inside me clicked, and I felt a tremendous peace that I knew would last.

Although intense emotion does not seem to be essential for a quantum change to occur or to exert a lasting effect, the emotional impact of an insightful quantum change can be quite powerful. Sometimes, in fact, it seems to the quantum changer to lie at the very heart of what has happened, as illustrated in this story:

The Flood

This happened to me fifteen years ago. My wife and I had been married for ten years, and we didn't have children and the biological clock was ticking. We hadn't tried to have children. There was school to finish, and then careers to get started, but now it was time, if we were ever going to have a family. We had sort of gone back and forth on it, and sometimes we were a little more positive, and sometimes we leaned away from having kids, but it hadn't been real because it was out there somewhere in the future. Now she was feeling the longing to be a mother, and I was dragging my feet. I had a hundred reasons why it wasn't a good idea.

I had an unusual opportunity that year. This wasn't the experience itself, just a prelude. I had been part of a men's support group seven years earlier in another city, and we got really close. We got to the place where we could say just about anything to each other, and we trusted each other. I knew I would be back in the city for a few days, and so I asked if we might have a reunion of the men who were still around. Quite a few still were, and it was great to see the guys again. We went around the room, taking turns as we did before, telling what was happening in our lives and what our current issues were. When it came my turn, I talked about this decision we were struggling with and how hard it was. "Are you still dealing with that issue?" They rudely reminded me that I had been talking about this a lot seven years before. "What is it about having kids that scares you most?" one of them asked.

"I guess it isn't really that there is any one thing I don't like," I said. "It's just that I don't really feel any positive draw to have kids. I don't really like children that much. I just don't have those feelings."

"Bullshit!" said the man next to me, at whose home we were meeting. He was a fairly gentle and soft-spoken fellow, and it startled me. "What was the first thing you did when you came in here?"

I thought about it. They had two adorable grade schoolers whom I had gotten to know during previous visits. They were just turning in, and I had gone back to say good night, tell them a story, and tuck them in. "Why did you do that?" he asked.

Tears came. I realized in that moment that I had created a cover story that I didn't like children. The truth was that at any gathering with adults and children, you'd be likely to find me on the floor with the kids. "But," I insisted, "I still don't really want to have my own. I wonder why that is."

Now, I need to say a little about my own childhood here. I have no complaints about it. We were poor, but I never really thought that much about it. There was just so much love there. My mother was an incredibly warm woman, and I adored my grandfather. We lived in his house. My earliest memory is of a game we played when I was small. I would stand at one end of the hall and my parents would stand at the other end hugging, and I would run down the hall and snuggle in between them where it was all warm and loving. Anyhow, when I was five, my sister was born, and we were close. When she was four or five, maybe, she was diagnosed with childhood diabetes, and when she was eight years old, she died suddenly on Easter Sunday. We were devastated. It took me a long time to work through my grief about that, and I still have some, of course, but we had some amazing pastors who helped me through it. I had also worked on it in therapy and was pretty sure that losing her did not really explain my lack of interest in having kids.

I haven't said much about my father. My memory of him was as a sad, depressed, lonely, withdrawn, and distant man. There was no doubt that he loved us. He worked on the railroad his entire life to provide for us, and it was hard, cold, brutal labor. When he came home at night, he was exhausted. He was just not there really—tired, melancholy, bitter. It was as if the winters had frozen his spirit.

One night my wife and I were sitting on the couch, again talking about children. I guess I was saying something about not feeling any desire for children myself and listening to her longing. All of a sudden, I was just flooded with memories. It happened in an instant, just like that. It wasn't like watching a movie. It was more like downloading files on a computer; it happened that fast. What I got back were vivid memories of how my father had been before my sister died. He had been playful, funny, energetic. He would romp on the floor with us. He wrestled with us and tickled us and told us stories. He had an old shortwave radio that could pull in amazing things from all over the world, and we would cuddle up and listen together.

I couldn't speak. I was just sobbing, sobbing, gasping for

breath. It must have been ten minutes before I could say anything at all. I would try to say a word and just break down weeping again. My wife held me and waited until I could explain.

In that moment, I realized what had happened. When I lost my sister, I also lost my father. It killed him. He lived for another fifteen years, but it killed him emotionally right then. What I had been remembering before as my father was only how he had been after her death, when I was a teenager. What came back to me was all of the loving memories of him before that terrible day. I still weep, because I feel for that man. All those years of so much pain, buried so deep. And I knew what had happened. Somewhere inside I had made a decision that anything that could do that to a man, I wanted no part of. It terrified me. It wasn't losing my sister so much as seeing how it destroyed my father, just tore him apart from us and from life.

That part of me healed in that moment. I understood. As an adult, I could separate my father's pain from myself. It's quite something, how my mind had just walled off those feelings, letting me still experience them while also denying them. After that, I no longer feared being destroyed by the love I felt for children. It was OK to feel it. The dam broke, and the tears flowed, and parts of my soul that had been isolated were reunited.

We have two children now, and they have children. I have learned so much from them and from being a father and grandfather. It's amazing how much pain and anxiety you can feel as a parent. I had never experienced such intense emotions, and I drew on everything I had ever learned, and a lot of prayer, too, to make it through. But pain is just the other side of love. They come together as a package. We feel pain when we care, because we care. That's just the way we're made.

Knowledge

It is a frequent feature of both insightful and mystical quantum changes that one has the experience of receiving new knowledge or truth. Often it is knowledge about oneself, and sometimes it has the quality of larger truth as well. It is an interesting feature that this insight comes with an immediate certainty of its veracity. For some it is a reasonably circumscribed realization, while others are given, in the words of Fools Crow quoted at the start of this chapter, "a great deal of knowledge in a brief period of time. It is a powerful experience that almost overwhelms you." There can be a sense of immediate *recognition*, as if somehow one already knew it to be true. One man described an "instantaneous and fearsome" moment of quantum change in which a new reality hit him like a lightning bolt:

> *The whole thing came together for me, where I realized that there is a universal whole and through it I'm tied to you and to everything in the universe. I saw that there's something much greater than this physical world that we live in, and I started asking, "What is real, what is the meaning of life, what should I strive for?" I realized that what was in my mind had been distorted, that as a kid I was formed into something that my natural self wasn't. It hit me that I was tied together with all those people I had crunched and bulldozed along the way, and that being kind to them was superimportant.*

Control

There seem to be some common themes to quantum change insights. A frequent theme is control.[13] Sometimes the insight has to do with the need to stop trying to control and instead to accept that which is beyond personal control. Sometimes it has to do with relinquishing control by "turning it over" to someone else or to a Higher Power.[14] And sometimes quantum change involves realizing the need and ability to *take* control and responsibility for one's life. All of these have something to do with gaining a greater grasp of one's place in the universe. One man's description of his quantum change included this insight:

> *I realized that I could set myself free from my past and really live now, that I could choose at any moment in time how I feel. . . . What's in my mind really is my choice. I never had seen it that way before. I'd always been a victim. . . . What I knew in that moment is that it was me.*

Another such observation came from a woman with lupus, a chronic and somewhat unpredictable disorder of the body's connective tissue. She had suffered long, and after one particularly frustrating day in which she felt dismissed and patronized by her physicians, she wrote them off:

I knew that day with absolute certainty that things were going to be different. It just felt different from all the half-hearted resolutions I had ever made in my life. I knew for sure that if doctors can't help me, then I'm going to have to do it myself, and that is what I did, starting from that day up to now. The biggest change was taking control, believing that I knew more about myself and my body than anybody else, and now two years later, I'm feeling the best that I have felt in at least ten years.

An interesting aspect of insightful quantum changes is that they usually alter much more than the particular area of the person's life that seemed to trigger them. In this woman's case, the focus of the insight was on taking responsibility for her own health care in regard to the lupus, but the effects of the insight pervaded broad areas of her life, including her relationships with family and friends, and her sense of herself as a person.

In the final chapter of this book, we will explore these common insights that emerge from quantum change experiences.

THE STORIES THAT FOLLOW

In sum, the insightful type of quantum change seems to center on a grand "aha," an awareness that breaks on the shores of consciousness with tremendous force. To the person experiencing one of these, it is clear that this is no ordinary insight or decision. It comes like a lightning bolt, and the profound truth of it is immediately and stunningly evident. The experience itself is often quite emotional, ultimately leaving a sense of peacefulness and resolution. They are highly memorable moments and constitute an abrupt turning point in the person's life.

Each of the next five chapters presents a detailed first-hand account of an insightful quantum change. We chose these particular interviews because they illustrate so well not only the basic nature of the insightful type, but also some other common aspects of quantum change in general. As life experiences, they sound less dramatic than Scrooge's story and the epiphanies recounted in Part III. Yet for those who experienced them, these quantum changes were dramatic turning points in life.

The first of these five experiences (Chapter 5) began after a counseling session, while a woman was driving home in her truck. Her "boom" has the quality of an emotional cleansing or catharsis, and she describes the "seeing" aspect of an insightful quantum change that was, for her, the beginning of an ongoing process of searching.

In contrast, the next storyteller (Chapter 6) had been quite content with her life. The "train" that blindsided her was an unexpected encounter with a guru. Like the man "on the island" at the beginning of this chapter, she was searching for a way to help others but wound up being transformed herself. For her it was no single insight, but a rush of truth. She describes in more detail the aftermath of her experience.

A sequence of events involving a mirror and two roses became turning points for a young man who had been wandering aimlessly through life (Chapter 7). He offers a more detailed account of the events leading up to a quantum change, and as a fitting symbol, his precursor events occurred on the eve of a new year. His story illustrates an interesting aspect of some quantum change experiences: he took a series of actions, with no conscious idea why he was doing so. As will be illustrated later, in Part III, some quantum changers experience this as their own will having been superseded for a short period of time. Others experience it as subtle guidance, and still others remain puzzled as to why they did what they did. It led this young man to a moment of convergence, an act that left him with a dramatic peacefulness and a new sense of himself.

The storyteller of "Awakening" (Chapter 8) had a similar experience, suddenly and inexplicably knowing a profound calmness and finding a wholly new perception of herself. She, too, had been drifting, not consciously searching, when she was caught up in the rapids. She describes well the startling suddenness and finality of this knowing, and how it differs from coming to a conclusion rationally. The content of her insight is not readily described in words, as particular principles or facts that she came to see. Rather, it was a different way of seeing and an utterly transformed awareness of the seer.

The last of these five insight stories (Chapter 9) comes from one who had been wandering aimlessly. After seven years she wandered into a Buddhist community in Tibet and came face to face with a life-changing moment of choice. Her account highlights an element of decision that some quantum changers describe—of being able to say yes or no to the experience, to accept or reject it.

What is common to all five of these stories is a sudden insightful awakening, a crystallization of awareness. All of these storytellers were taken by surprise; and in one day they all passed through a doorway that they would never see again.

5

BOOM

There was a social worker who was a friend of mine because we worked together. One morning when riding to work with him, I told him that I thought I was a little bit obsessive. When we got to work he showed me a book called the DSM (the *Diagnostic and Statistical Manual of Mental Disorders*). It has all of the personality disorders and little grey boxes with the symptoms of each one. I'd never seen it or heard of it before, so he started showing me the diagnostic symptoms of the obsessive-compulsive.

I said, "Well, I used to do that a little bit, and I do this, but I don't do this and I don't do that." I'm not at all compulsive, and it didn't seem to fit. Then he flipped it over to the narcissistic personality, because I'd been complaining to him about problems with my marriage. I read the symptoms of narcissistic personality and said, "My God! This is my husband. He does every one of the symptoms on the list. What is this book? Let me borrow it!"

I read the whole section on personality disorders, and my husband fit the criteria for four personality disorders, plus maybe two more. So the next day at work the director was in my office, and I asked him about personality disorders, but he said he didn't know much and I should ask a psychologist. Just then a counselor walked past my door, so I stopped him and asked if people who have personality disorders ever get better. It seemed to me like he stood there for a long time. He was leaning against the door jamb, and then he slowly shook his head no, and I said, "I have to get a divorce."

Now, this same counselor was our employee assistance person. I went to him for free, and it was kind of interesting therapy because it wasn't at all what I thought it would be.

I got very frustrated with it, trying to do it his way. He just kept telling me I was wrong every time I was right. I think now that what I needed was a good listener, instead of what he was doing. He talked me into coming into town as a private patient, and there was something wrong with that whole relationship too.

I had known him at work and we were actually kind of friends, but I stayed with it thinking that it must be me who didn't know and that the therapist knew the answers. I kept going to this counselor for support, but that's not exactly what I got.

Finally one day I had just finished our session. I stood up to leave, and I don't know what triggered it, but this horrendous emotional thing started happening to me. It's hard to describe, because it's like you suddenly see everything at once. It just goes "boom" like that, and then the emotions start coming up. It's like it came up from my feet and all up my body, and I knew something was happening. I knew I was going to cry or something, so I told him, "I have to get out of here," and headed down the hall. He asked, "Are you mad at me?" and I said, "Hell no, I'm not mad at you!"

Now this is all very out of character for me to do that. I got out the door and into my truck and drove home.

I saw through tears all the way home. I guess it's about three miles and I must have used fifteen Kleenexes. I tend not to be a cryer. I'm always shocked when I read those statistics about how often people cry a week or a month or whatever. When I cry, it's usually at what I feel is appropriate. It has to do with me, when I feel it, and not because the culture says it's OK to cry at that time. I just tend not to cry a lot, and this was sobbing, just sobbing.

When I got home, I went out on the back patio, the small backyard of the house, and I just railed at the world. It was one of those July days, late in the afternoon, probably six or seven, where the thunderstorm is coming, the black clouds are rolling in, and there's lightning off in the distance. I was swearing and yelling, being very loud, which again is out of character for me. I guess the thunder and rain would cover it as far as the neighbors could tell. I had no idea what it was, or what it was going to be. I just allowed it to happen. I didn't stop it, because I think you can stop those things.

After this explosion happened I really went searching. I wanted to know what this was. The main thing that happened to me after that explosion was this inner peace. All that horrendous emotion came out, and there was inner peace. I was asking questions. I went back to Judeo-Christianity and traced it clear back. I started asking, "What is this that is called God? Where did that come from historically?" My mind was just rolling. I began to see that there's this inner connectedness, which is what real reality is all about.

My whole life started changing.

It's hard to explain. It's like in a flash you can see everything at once. Everybody sees something different when this happens, because it has to come from what you have experienced and know, what you name, so each person sees something different. It changed the basis of how I perceive, opened up my eyes. Your perception is your reality. It's your truth.

6

TAKING THE AA TRAIN

I still refer to my experience as being hit by a freight train. It was the Truth with a capital T, and it was really quite overwhelming. It was exciting, but it was also very painful and shocking and tearful. I remember the next morning I got up and promptly threw up. I felt like I had the flu, but I didn't. It was just so powerful that all the stuff I was assimilating hit me like a ton of bricks. I knew it was the truth. I recognized it when I heard it.

I'd been around it all these years, thirteen years in the Alcoholics Anonymous (AA) program, and heard bits and pieces of it, but finally I heard the truth clearly and concisely presented. This is what the original AA program was—a very truthful, spiritual concept.

I've been in AA for almost fourteen years now, and in that period I have had good progress in recovery and working the AA program. Still, I was having some difficulties with some people I was sponsoring, and so about a year ago I thought, "I'll call this person who's teaching the Big Book and ask for advice." I had come in contact with some friends who were having really good results in their working of the program in that they were connecting more with the spiritual part of it in a way that they hadn't been able to before. They told me about a class that was being taught on the Big Book of AA that was very thorough and helped people get the essential message of the Big Book. I was skeptical that one person teaching a class could get this message across any more clearly than anyone reading this book on his or her own could. So I was a little uneasy contacting him. I had heard so many emotional, profound reactions to the way he had helped other people. I was thinking, "Oh, come on; this is a little too much. This guy sounds like one of these gurus."

But once we were on the phone, he referred again and again to the Big Book for answers that were incredibly clear, precise, accurate, and right on the nail as far as what was really going on with me and the people I was trying to assist. These were people with new recovery, new to sobriety, trying to keep a grip on it. The clarity and truthfulness of his help was just astonishing to me. He said a lot of things that were the opposite of what was being taught in AA. He referred to specific lines of pages just right off the top of his head, which was really amazing. I thought the way he answered my questions using this information, the way he knew the Big Book, was just pretty mind boggling. It shook me up. It really shook me up. I said, "Well, thank you," and concluded the phone call.

About half an hour later he called back and said, "If you'd like me to take you through the first part of the book, maybe what I can teach you in a few hours could help this person you're working with and you can pass it on."

It ended up being five hours. It seemed like twenty minutes. He was so precise, intense, and exact in answering all my questions, and I was full of questions. I was to leave the next day on a plane, but within that five hours of going over the Big Book, I experienced just a complete transformation of my understanding, not only of the AA program but of my view of the world, my whole outlook on life.

I wasn't drinking coffee that day, but I felt highly energized. I just felt like if I drank coffee I'd blow off the face of the earth. I was already real hyped energywise. There was this adrenaline of my mind embracing and consuming this material that I'd been hungry for for a long time. I was crying for joy. I really wanted to know this stuff. It was just like I knew it when I heard it, I recognized it. I was really exhilarated—extremely, cheerfully happy that I'd finally found what I'd been looking for.

I went away kind of in a stupor for the rest of that day. I ended up taking study tapes home with me and listened to those. Over the following months I proceeded to study the Big Book more, learn more, and be more effective as a recovering alcoholic. I *became* a recovering alcoholic, whereas before, even though I was sober, I had

had emotional ups and downs, roller coasters, anger that was out of control, and just a lot of still sick behavior.

Now I was completely blown out of the water. I saw that there absolutely was nothing but doom ahead for me if I didn't do certain things that provided certainty and hope. I had gone to this person feeling like I had all these years of sobriety. I had all this experience. I had worked with all these people. My little life was just great. I didn't think I needed anything to happen. I wasn't going because I was distraught or anything. I was just looking for some good ideas to help the people I was sponsoring. That's really all I expected. I went there to look for solutions for other people, and I found a solution for myself.

I was completely devastated, but it was a joyful sort of devastation because I saw the solution within the same period of seeing the doom. In all my years of searching for solutions I had studied lots of different faiths and religions, philosophies of the world, and dabbled in the occult. I realized that this was essential truth that pulled together all the truths of all the great religions and philosophers. You know, there are so many denominations around and millions of people saying, "Our way is the only way." Now I have that sense of unity above it all and what the world is really about. That made it even more powerful to me, because I knew that this thread ran through everything else that was of value.

I've seen other people get blown away. Almost everybody who's worked with this person has had this experience. Some people don't get it. Some people reject it or don't want to hear it, but generally people get reawakened. What you learn is complete reliance on God. I'd had glimpses of relying on God in my life, but never so totally.

I've tried to explain to my husband what happened, and he's seen the change. He saw me just being nicer and sweeter and happier, at least more of the time. I used to be kind of glum and depressing. I'm just happier. He'd noticed through the years that I'd lost a lot of my cheerfulness of our early years, and now more of my spirit has come back. He said how wonderful he thinks some of these changes are, but he just has no idea what's gone on. That's kind of sad to me, because I love him deeply. We've been married a long time. I'd like him to know, but he's in a good place. It's not like he needs to go through the same experience I've been through.

My interest in things I was previously interested in has really dropped off. Things I used to do for entertainment or just to pass the time seem totally aimless now. I used to find it relaxing to go to the malls and walk around and maybe go shopping. I lost interest in most things for a while. I'm getting back an interest in gardening, cooking, but for a while everything dropped away. Everything else seemed totally meaningless besides working with Big Book stuff. Now I think I'm getting more balance. I still find that sitting and looking through a fashion magazine doesn't have the appeal it used to. It's like I'm wasting time. There is so much to be done, and I've got the energy to do it, so I should do it, the good stuff.

The experience of becoming more effective as a recovering alcoholic just kept right on happening the more I listened to the book, the more I read the book, but not everything has changed. I'm still hyper. I'm still real talkative. I still have some trouble with my temper, though it's much better. That's something I've been praying, working on getting some results with. I still like my home and my family. There was a brief time where I thought I might even just leave everything and go off and do this teaching stuff, but that's not a wise decision. I'm very committed to my family. I work with other people in the AA program more, so there have been some demands on my family in terms of more childcare. I'm gone more than I used to be, and so I'm trying right now to balance that out. But I think the kids are better off. I'm a better mother. I'm able to devote more time to feeling comfortable with my role in my home as well as this working with others, whereas before I was a lot more restless. I was doing it, but I was really restless. I'm content to be home and to do what is before me that I know I need to do. I've never been a heavy person, but I became real aware of how I used food to gratify me. Now I'm just working on my spiritual life and getting in contact with what God wants me to do, and then that gratification stuff goes away.

Before, I used to schedule my days pretty tightly. Now I don't plan way ahead on events or scheduling because I know that I get up and I do what I need to do. I get my kids off to school, and the day just sort of unfolds as it should. Phone calls might start coming in, or I might need to work with a person in the afternoon, or some homeless lady comes to my door. Some really interesting things just unfold out of the day. I know to trust that the day will unfold. I don't have to be scurrying all over doing eight thousand things to keep

myself entertained or active. I trust that what I need to do next will
be right in front of me, will be real obvious.

My friends are still my friends. I've tried to explain to a few of
them what I've gone through, and they've been interested and supportive. I'm more open about my involvement with AA than I used
to be. I used to tell certain friends that I was in AA, but now I just
tell everybody what I do and why I do it. I have a total comfort with
what I am supposed to be doing. In these last few months I have
been neglecting my regular friends because I do all this other work,
and I realized that I can't do that. That's not a good idea. There has to
be a balance, but my good friends have stayed my good friends. I've
always had good, close, personal relationships, and I've made more
friends because of the work I'm doing with these other people. I feel
like I've been able to be of help to many of my friends because now
that I'm more open with what I do, they inevitably have a mother or
an uncle or somebody who's in some kind of recovery. I also do more
service within my church now. I see more clear signs of where I can
be of help now, rather than just occasionally baking cookies. I feel
more sensitive to how I can be of service. That's what I'm trying to
say! I'm trying to be aware of where my time can best be spent in service to others.

Now I use my faith in God to guide me for everything. I'm practicing, learning more and more to pray every day about everything.
It must sound so corny to say that, but it's true. I'm learning to trust
in God's guidance. His guidance, the guidance of my Higher Power,
is right and true. It's never wrong, so the more I can keep in touch
with that, the better off my life is out here.

My optimism is growing in terms of what's really happening in
the world and in humankind. I think we're on an upward spiral of
growth. I think things are getting better. I know the world has terrible problems, but my worldview now is that things are moving upward compared to twenty years ago, three hundred years ago, a
thousand years ago. Before I thought that things were just so bad,
that crime was so bad and the world was so sick, with so many bad
things happening. Overall, there's a movement upward, I think. No,
I *believe* it. I don't think it.

I have a real secure feeling about the future. I just feel like
there'll be more of these good things happening. Good things *are*
happening. Good things *were* happening for me. It's hard to explain

this. I had quite a good life, but it's getting even better. I just have faith that I'm going in real good directions. It's hard work, it's stressful, but it's good. It's hard to describe it in any other way but that it's good and right and true. When I learned not to rely on my own directing and controlling things all the time, life became much more harmonious. I'm learning to trust in my Higher Power and not to be afraid.

7

A MIRROR AND TWO ROSES

I grew up in a small town up in the mountains of New Mexico. We moved away from there when I was fourteen, which is the year my mother died. In high school I got straight A's, but I never dated and was something of a loner. I always tried to fade into the woodwork and not be noticed. Then while I was at the university, my father died, just six years after my mother. I started having panic attacks, and at first I didn't know what they were. I called an ambulance once to take me to the hospital because I thought I was having a heart attack.

It was hard for me to go to school after that. I was not very happy. I didn't know what I wanted. I didn't really like school. I was having a pretty rough time personally as well as academically, so I decided I'd better quit school, get my act together, and find out what I want, who I am.

That was a low period of my life. I guess you would say I hit rock bottom. I had a lack of confidence, a really poor self-image. I was very unhappy, very depressed. I didn't like myself. I didn't like other people. During that time I guess my pattern was to get up in the morning, go to work, buy a six-pack, come home, drink until I passed out, and get up again the next morning. I wouldn't say I drank every single day or every single night. It's just that that's what I would do—I'd just go home and be alone. I was financially in the hole, and I lived in a hellhole.

This whole thing started one day when a friend I hadn't seen for several years walked into the place where I was working and just about freaked out when he saw me. He looked at me and said, "You're fat!" Now this sounds hilarious, but no one had ever told me that before and it was not my self-image at all. I thought, "How dare you tell me that? I'm not fat! Who are you to tell me that?" It sounds like such an insignificant incident, but it was like someone was telling me something about myself that I didn't know. It felt very significant, because it meant I didn't even know who I was! That was the first of three events that led up to this.

On New Year's Eve that year I was feeling particularly depressed. I packed a bag and got into my car, not really knowing where I was going. I went downtown to a hotel and checked into a room. I bought a bottle of bourbon and just hung out in that room all day and overnight. The second significant thing happened when I got up the next day. I was packing to check out when I looked in the mirror. I didn't recognize what I saw. There was a real split, I guess, between my inner self and the self that the outside world could see. I didn't like what I saw. I saw a fat person. I saw someone who looked like he was experiencing some physical deterioration due to alcohol. I didn't see a healthy person. I didn't see a happy person. I guess that's really what it all boils down to. It woke me up.

I decided at that point, "My life is shot to hell. There's got to be something that I can do. I've got to accomplish something. I've got to prove to myself I'm worth something and I can do something: set a goal, make a plan, and meet that plan." So I just sat down and thought, "You're a smart person. What can you do to make yourself feel better?"

I had never exercised regularly, but I started walking every day. Then I began running. After a year I was still at it, running six miles at least twice a week. I also started eating healthier foods, and it worked. I slimmed down, and people noticed and complimented me. I stopped drinking heavily. During the same time I began feeling more confident and taking initiative in the business where I worked. My ideas were successful for the company, and within the year they had doubled my salary. I moved to a nicer apartment and bought a new car.

It was then, exactly one year after I looked in the mirror on New

Year's Eve, that the most dramatic thing happened. I was in my new apartment, and I decided I wanted to test-drive my new car. It was like my old pattern—let's just go out and do something. I decided I wanted to go to the town where I had grown up. I knew I was going to be gone for probably a couple of days, so I packed some luggage. I hadn't been back there in seven years, since my father had died. I wasn't comfortable actually going to see people I knew. I just wanted to drive into town, drive around, and reminisce. So I shot up there late in the afternoon and checked into a hotel on New Year's Eve. I just stayed in the room, so I didn't really celebrate the New Year. I contemplated going down to the bar, but I said, "Nah, I don't feel like it."

I got up early the next morning and drove to a lake outside town. It's really interesting how your perception of time changes between when you're growing up and when you're an adult. I remember going to that lake when I was a kid, and it seemed like it took hours, at least an hour to drive there. In reality, it took me about twelve minutes. Then I drove back down into town. I just drove all over. I drove to see the house I grew up in and went to check out some of the old neighbors' houses. I checked on all my schools there. I just drove around, stopping the car and checking things out. It was funny, because things had not really changed at all. I drove downtown. I walked the main street. The main drag is three or four blocks long, three or four street lights—that's about it. A lot of the stores had changed or closed. They went through real hard times financially, that little town, so it's a pretty depressed place.

Finally I did what I had to do. I stopped at a florist shop, bought two red roses, got in the car, and drove to the cemetery. It was seven years later, but I knew exactly where to go. I went to the graves, and I just stood there for a while and talked to my parents. I told them I was doing much better and I missed them, and I cried. That's when the big thing hit.

It was like this cloud just lifted, like this calm and serenity settled in. I felt good. I felt happy for the first time in over a decade, since I was fourteen, when my mother died. At that point it finally hit me. This was the first time I had ever said good-bye to my parents. It wasn't really a religious thing, like people who are born again. I'm not a religious person. I understand a lot of people say they go through dramatic changes with religious connotations. That wasn't really the case with me.

I was there maybe an hour. It was funny, too, because I had been listening to this tape and just as I was driving out of the cemetery this song came on, "Good-bye, Good-bye." It was just so perfect. It was perfect.

That was five years ago, and it's stayed with me until this very day. It was really a dramatic thing. It's as if very shortly after that I found out who I was, and who I am, and what I want. I found myself. I'm just about to finish up my degree, and I plan to open my own business. I like myself now. I like life. I like everything. I try to get as much as I can out of every day. I want to know that I have lived this day as fully as I could. The depression is gone, and that feeling of wanting to fade into the woodwork is gone, too. I'm not afraid to approach other people. I can't say that I'm perfect. I've grown a lot. I've matured a lot. I still sometimes feel a sense of anxiety, I guess—a sense of fear—but it's not nearly as strong as it was before. I know that everybody during the course of a day has some fear in some situations. I think that's just normal.

From that point on, it was like I was experiencing things for the first time in my life. I've had some incredible experiences, and it's been great. I've become close to a lot of people. I'm very close to my sister, and I have a very close friend I'm dating. I guess that after going through one experience like this, one thing just starts building on top of the other. It gets better and better, where everything gets easier and easier. I feel I can do just about anything I want. I feel that I control my life; life doesn't control me anymore. There's just this inner strength in me. I knew it was there, but I had never been able to tap it. Now it's there, and it's getting stronger all the time.

8

AWAKENING

Exactly how it happened is still somewhat of a mystery to me. I had been married for almost twenty years. The marriage was satisfactory but never really happy. Then one day I suddenly felt a sense of presence about myself that I had never felt before. I knew that the way I was living was not right—that there was more, and most important that there was more to me. I had been living a part of myself, but a part that was a hazy sort of person who moved through life and did things well, without a strong awareness or consciousness.

That one day, I just became very aware of this. I just felt this presence of a real self within me. I had always thought that I knew who I was, but that afternoon, I really felt the body that I had been given and the person, the soul that was in this body. Before, whichever way life went, I went along with it and did the best I could. Now, all of a sudden, I had a sense of myself, that I had a specific course to take, and I couldn't meander any longer.

It seems like it happened in a flash, and then that was it. There was no turning back. There was no more room for "Oh, well, I'll try this scheme for a while. I'll try this and see if maybe this will make my life a little better." It just wiped everything clean, like a wake-up call, but not a harsh one. It was more a feeling, or a presence—somewhere in between there. I felt alive in every space of my body, that I was aware of every bit of space that my body was. It wasn't so much a sensation, like a tingling or something like that. It was more a solidness, but the solidness wasn't in my mind, like "Boy, everything's going to be good" or "This is what's going to happen now." It was more that I knew that I am more than what I thought I was. I felt whole, and the wholeness contained every part of my body. No matter what could happen at that moment—a hurricane or anything—I would have a sense of OK-ness, a sense that everything was all right. The entire universe was all right.

Everything had a calmness to it. My life had been in such an agitated, chaotic state for so many years that I wasn't aware of how out of balance, how crazy I was living my life until this experience happened. All of that left, the agitation left, and I just felt this soothing comfort, a quietness. And everything—like my children and my household—seemed to be brighter. There seemed to be a brightness, a kind of clarity, as if a fog had been lifted. A film that had covered everything was gone.

I see it as an act of grace. I had been doing transcendental meditation for almost fifteen years. I guess there wasn't any other way that I was going to get the message. I had eighteen years of a pretty sad life, not even realizing how sad it was. There were all the messages, all the knock-knocks that came, but I just was not willing to receive them. I look back now, and I see that I was barricading the door. When I knew somebody was knocking at the door and saying "Listen," I said, "No, no, no. I don't want to hear it." So it took a big kebang to get my attention.

I approached my husband and told him that my life wasn't right, that our marriage was not right, and that we had to do something about it. I mean tangibly we had to do something. We had to see a counselor. We had to start straightening out the course of our lives. He wasn't interested. He felt that our life was fine. I said, "We both know that it's not, and unless you're willing to participate in the change, it's over. This is finally going to be the end." He left three days later. The old part of me longed to just continue the way my life had been, the way I had been performing, but there was a stronger part of me. It almost seems like it came from the back of me. It was like a presence that was stronger than the smaller part of me that had been ruling my life, and it was moving me toward this specific path that I had entered.

I'm still not exactly sure what that path is other than awareness that this world and I are not simply physical. It's just something that I felt and I saw very clearly, and once I saw it, that was it. I couldn't forget it. It was a clarity that was so real. There was no negotiating with my husband, or maybe more important, there was no negotiating with me. This is what my life was, and I had to take responsibility for that for myself.

I have found, and I'm still finding, that I have to get out of the way of myself. When I try to take control and I think "This is what I need to do," I find that I'm veering off. I need to move out of the way and more just feel myself in my heart. It's much harder, being responsible, feeling not only responsible for myself but feeling a responsibility toward the whole earth. Sometimes I wish I could just fall back into that foggy type of perception that I had about everything. Before, I just felt powerless, like there was nothing I could do about suffering in the world.

With this awareness it's a lot of real hard work, and I find a lot of sadness in it, too. Things bother me so much more now. I'm hoping that I come to a point where when I see homeless people or I see kids who are having problems, street kids, instead of feeling so burdened and saddened by it, I'll be in a position to be able to act, to do something about it. I'd like to be more of a living force, to see it as it is and be able to do something about it. I used to think, "There are other people who do that, those people out there," and now I see that I *am* those people. There is no such thing as "those people." They are us, me. It's each individual, and I guess that's where the burden is that I feel. There is no designated group of people who are placed on the earth to do good works. It's each of us. That's where I am right now, realizing that I do have the ability, that I do have the power, that I do have the responsibility to do something about it.

I know that there is something I'm destined to do, that there is a greater purpose for me. That doesn't mean I am going to move the earth or do something profound, but it is profound in the sense that I have found my place on earth. I have made that connection with God. I'm just a person walking around here on earth. God is within me, and I have to pay more attention to the godliness that is really truly me. There's something specific that I'm here for.

I used to see everybody and everything as either good or bad, right or wrong. Now there really isn't any right and there isn't any wrong. I had real problems with that—I mean that's one of my biggest anguishes about this whole thing. I deal with it daily. It's real difficult to be angry with anything that's occurring in the world, because it's all happening for a reason. I am in no position to judge anything. Just see it as it is, and if there's something that I can do to help elevate a person's awareness, that's what I hope I can do. I feel a lot more tender toward people, in contrast with how I isolated myself before. It's a kind of a sweetness that I feel for people. I don't feel separate, like "That's them and this is me." It's just us. There really isn't any separation there at all.

I find I grow very impatient with small talk. I don't like gossipy stuff. I don't like chitchat, just to be talking. Sitting in silence in a room with somebody would be more comfortable for me than to have to talk to one another just because we're in the same room or just to be talking. I've taken a good look at my friendships. I cherish the ones that are real connections with people and have let other ones go. I still enjoy my friendships that are more on a surface level, but they're not important to me any longer. I found that the specialness of friendships, the quality of communication and connectedness you have with another person, is a real special thing, and I think there's something divine when you connect with somebody in a real way. Romantic friendships have become less and less important, and I know that's because I'm letting go of the romantic notion of love. I'm finding in myself what love really is, and romantic love now seems silly or superficial.

If I think of the future at all, I think of the future in terms of God, of joining with God, and with the godliness within me. I don't see the future as something out there like great wealth, or being famous, or some grand discovery in science. I'm so focused on each day, on what I'm doing each day and trying to be aware of each minute, that it doesn't leave a lot of time for projecting myself into the future.

I see my spirituality as just that, my spirituality. I've read a lot of the old mystics and saints and so forth. My intention in reading these books when I started out was to try to find a way. I see now that nobody can give me a way. We each have our own individual path toward self-actualization, toward enlightenment. People can give you ideas, or for me it's more like I connect with something that somebody has said, and I recognize it, and I say "Oh, yes!" It's almost like little beacons of light, little signs or guideposts along the way. I can't look *out there* anymore for my way to fulfillment because I know it's all within me.

9

RIPPLES

I was raised in Texas, in a very small town. I was always a very rebellious, nonstereotypical girl for my age. Oh, I enjoyed all the silly things that young girls do, but when I was younger I would rather play Tarzan than Jane. I have always been very aggressive. I was always a leader. Once I got through high school, I went through an intense rebellious period. I was a radical in the civil rights movement, and I protested against the war in Vietnam as a member of Students for a Democratic Society. I was a heroin addict, too. I just did a lot of things. I crammed an intense amount of experiences into my life, and I was not dedicated to any one thing. It was "Run over here and do this for a while, and then run over there."

At one point during my drug addiction, I realized that I needed to be a little more purposeful, whatever that was, and I quit heroin myself, cold turkey. I got away from drugs and friends who did drugs. I got away from friends who were very radical and from protest groups and was just with myself. That's when I began getting the idea that it would be very important for me to travel, not doing anything specific but just being open to what might reveal itself. I traveled around Europe for four or five months and spent some time in North Africa and followed the overland hippie trail through Turkey, Iran, Afghanistan, and Pakistan to India. I can't really say at this time that I was looking to hit a spiritual chord in myself, but when I went

into Nepal I met a fellow who thought I might connect to Eastern religious practice. He told me he had heard that there was a Tibetan
lama in a little village outside of Katmandu and that maybe I should
see him.

It took some time, but I found the place, and at that time the
center wasn't well developed at all. There were maybe eighty West-
erners there, and the meditation sessions were held in a large tent. It
was very primitive conditions, and we followed monastic rules,
which was really a change for me, having been living such a foot-
loose and fancy-free life for nearly seven years. We awoke at 4:30 in
the morning and took tea, then went in for the first meditation session at 5:30. At 6:30 we had a meal and then teachings in the morning. There was a meal before noon, which was the only main food we
had each day. After the meal there was a rest period, and then more
teachings and questions and answers in the afternoon, then tea and
usually two to three more hours of meditation in the evening. All
this was done in silence for thirty days. [*She begins crying.*] I'm sorry.
It still affects me very strongly.

Of course, we all broke silence sometimes. It was such an intense time emotionally that there were just times when I had to cling
to someone, and had to talk and they had to talk about all the things
that were going on. We're so attached to the image and the entity of
"self," and to all the things we are that create that self. When you're
sitting there meditating, you have to confront that entity of self, all
of it: the positive parts and the negative parts and the neutral parts.
That's when I went through the change. I knew that if I was ever going to really uncover the best of me, some incredibly strong parts of
me had to be tempered or . . . I'm trying to think of the proper word
. . . they had to be redirected.

I think it's something that has to click very quickly, or you lose
the impetus to do it. As human beings, we are great rationalizers.
You have to strike while the iron is hot, so to speak, or you tend to
fall back into old habit patterns and rationalize why you do that. I
suddenly realized that this was what had to be done, and the change
I went through involved immediately striking. There's that little
thing, you know—for me it's like it's here in my chest area somewhere—that's always there throughout your life. You always know
when you're doing something that's right or not right, and it was really telling me that this was the right thing for me to do. I *knew* for
certain that I was taking the most important step of my life. I real-

ized right then that either I made a commitment or I left, because if I stayed a very important change was going to happen in my life. I knew that this was not some hocus-pocus, mumbo-jumbo bullshit, but that somebody was fixing to expose me to myself, and if I didn't want that exposure, I should leave. It's just very intense, it happens very quickly. You have to shut your mouth and look at yourself.

I knew that a certain amount of discipline was very important at this time in my life. I'd always had to be a disciplined person when I lived under the rules of my mother and my father, because they always had very strict rules and both of them were very disciplined people. Of course, part of my rebellion was against that discipline. So I decided, since I'd had six or seven years of being totally undisciplined, that maybe I would be disciplined for this one time. I just made myself sit and listen. When we had meditation sessions, I disciplined myself to sit through the whole meditation even though Western legs aren't meant to sit like that for very long. There's a certain amount of teaching in working through pain. Most of my life, I had always run away from any confrontation, whether it was external or internal confrontation. That's 99% of the reason I got into drug use, because I couldn't confront my internal beingness.

I look back on that incident as incredibly important. If you want to be well, and be aware, and be of service on this planet—regardless of what you were, regardless of whatever unkindness you might have perpetrated upon yourself or others—a time comes when you just have to say, right now, "I'm not going to do that anymore." Right now—it has to do with right now. That's how I quit smoking cigarettes, too, after smoking for thirty years. There's a time when you just have to say, "I'm not going to do that anymore." I guess that was the decision I made that day: "I'm going to see this through."

After those thirty days, I went and got a house in the mountains and took this break where I just meditated and read a few books and thought about what had happened to me. When you go in a door and you're one person, and you come out that door and you're another person, you need time to sit and look. I remember I read Carl Jung's *Memories, Dreams and Reflections* during this time, and there's a part where he says we have these veils between our conscious mind and subconscious mind, and that it's very important to create a space where we can see beyond those veils. That's kind of what happened—like ripping veils down and every once in a while getting a glimpse of what's behind them.

I had gone through life up until that time with a total lack of ethics. I was a totally immoral, unethical person. I didn't give a great deal of thought to other people's feelings, or their place in my life, or their relationship to me. Once I crossed that line of commitment, I was constantly confronted by my desires and greed, my unkindness and lack of equanimity, and by the importance of compassion, of doing the right thing. Everybody has to make their own rule that works best for them, but we also have to remember when we're making those inner rules that we are all interconnected. When you make a rule for yourself, or make a decision for yourself, you have to think how it's going to have a ripple effect out here. That's what I mean by developing an ethical nature. You're concerned more about the ripple effect that it's going to have, because you realize how interconnected all of us are. You can no longer think of yourself as an isolated person.

PART III

EPIPHANIES

10

THE MYSTICAL TYPE
OF QUANTUM CHANGE

My depression deepened unbearably and finally it
seemed to me as though I were at the bottom of the pit.
I still gagged badly on the notion of a Power greater
than myself, but finally, just for a moment, the last
vestige of my proud obstinacy was crushed. All at once
I found myself crying out, "If there is a God, let Him
show Himself! I am ready to do anything, anything!"
Suddenly the room lit up with a great white light. I was
caught up into an ecstasy which there are no words to
describe. It seemed to me, in the mind's eye, that I was
on a mountain and that a wind not of air but of spirit
was blowing. And then it burst upon me that I was a
free man.   —BILL WILSON[15]

Insightful quantum changes, while in many ways stunning,
are easier to comprehend within a traditional psychological framework than are the mystical type. Insights are more readily understood as a sudden consolidation of psychological processes that may
have been building for years. They fit more neatly within orderly
conceptions of the human psyche. Perhaps over time the pieces of
the puzzle were coming together until finally they burst into consciousness as a completed picture.

It is more of a stretch to understand rationally the mystical quantum changes contained in this section. Those who have experienced such transformations are themselves typically at a loss to explain them. These experiences are simply overwhelming. They flood the person's thinking and feeling processes in such an intense manner that it is as though the person is being redesigned. Dr. William Silkworth, quoted in *Alcoholics Anonymous* (the Big Book), called them "vital spiritual experiences" and "huge emotional displacements and rearrangements."[16]

QUALITIES OF A MYSTICAL EXPERIENCE

A head start in understanding this type of quantum change is found in studies of mystical experiences more generally. There is a voluminous literature on the subject. Writing a century ago, William James[17] described four general characteristics of mystical experiences:

1. *Ineffability.* They are experiences that are more like feelings than thoughts, and that defy expression in words. The person feels incapable of adequately conveying the experience through language.
2. *Noetic quality.* They are also experienced as providing new insight and revelation that is of great depth and significance. The knowledge has an odd sense of authority about it; the person *knows* its truth. They can have the quality of nonrational direct experiences of the essential nature of existence, both of oneself and of the world.
3. *Transiency.* They do not last long, usually not more than half an hour, before they fade.
4. *Passivity.* They are not experienced as being under personal willful control. Rather, there is a sense of one's own will being temporarily suspended and sometimes of being in the grip or embrace of a higher power.

Drawing from a variety of sources in his 1963 doctoral dissertation at Harvard University, Walter Pahnke, who was both a physician and a pastor, added the following common characteristics to James's list[18]:

5. *Unity.* They produce an internal and external sense of unity of oneself with one's environment
6. *Transcendence.* They convey a perspective of the timelessness of life, transcending the limits of space and time. They may produce a paradoxical experience of transcendence in which the person feels simultaneously "out of the body" and "in the body."
7. *Awe.* They produce a sense of awe or sacredness, a non-rational intuitive response to being in the presence of inspiring realities
8. *Positivity.* They yield deeply felt positive emotions usually described as joy, peace, love, and blessing
9. *Distinctiveness.* They are transient states of awareness, felt to be quite different from ordinary experience.

Although not all of these attributes are present in every story, the family resemblance is plain. Yet there are quantum changes that lack many of the attributes of a mystical experience, as evidenced by those we have characterized as the insightful type. It is also the case that not all mystical experiences yield permanent and pervasive changes in the person. Some are experienced, make an immediate impression, but then fade away, leaving the person basically the same as before. "What was *that*?" one might ask after the first such mystical experience. Others are received simply as a blessing, an affirmation or confirmation, placing no demand upon the person. Paul Tillich[19] offered a classic description of this experience of acceptance:

> It is as though a voice were saying, "You are accepted, *you are accepted*, accepted by that which is greater than you, and the name of which you do not know. Do not ask for the name now; perhaps you will find it later. Do not try to do anything now; perhaps later you will do much. Do not seek for anything; do not intend anything. Simply accept the fact that you are accepted."

Perhaps the proper question is not why some mystical experiences induce permanent changes in people, but rather how so profound an experience could *fail* to produce a lasting effect. Abraham H. Maslow was particularly interested in mystical experiences and similar moments of elation and transcendence, giving them the term "peak experiences." Commenting on lasting positive changes that sometimes followed peak experiences, he wrote: "On the whole, these good aftereffects are easy enough to understand. What is more difficult to explain is the *absence* of discernible aftereffect in some people."[20] Sometimes the experience seems simply (yet profoundly) to confirm that the person is already on the right path. It is a memorable and often cherished experience, but not one that transforms the person's life.

It is also worth noting that there is some overlap between the characteristics of mystical experience and the general attributes of quantum change described in Chapter 2. Quantum change experiences are often ineffable, noetic, profoundly positive, and distinctive. Mystical experiences are often vivid and memorable, take one by surprise, and have a benevolent quality—all common characteristics of quantum change. Yet other characteristics that are typical of mystical experiences may or may not accompany a quantum change. Passivity, unity, transcendence, and awe—all described above as common elements of mystical experience—can be minimal or absent, particularly in the insightful type of quantum change. It is also clear that quantum changes are not transient. To be sure, there is often an *acute* initial experience that begins abruptly and then recedes, though many quantum changers also say that their experience did not have an ending.

The point here is that mystical experiences, though often accompanied by strong emotions, do not appear to be either necessary or sufficient for a quantum change to occur. Sometimes the abrupt onset of a quantum change is unambiguously mystical in quality, but in other cases it is not. This is why we have described a mystical subtype of quantum change that is distinguishable both from the insightful type and from mystical experiences that are not associated with substantial life change.

ATTRIBUTES OF THE MYSTICAL TYPE OF QUANTUM CHANGE

We found the nine attributes listed above to be quite descriptive of the acute experience of the mystical type of quantum change. We revisit these attributes now, this time drawing on the words of those who directly experienced them. Examining the attributes closely helps to clarify both the similarities and distinctions of the mystical type from quantum changes in general and from mystical experiences that do not trigger quantum changes.

1. Ineffability

Quantum changes in general have an elusive, ineffable quality about them. People find them hard to express in words. This seems to be even more pronounced in the mystical type, where there is often an encounter with realities for which there are no adequate words. Over time, as the experience consolidates, people may find ways of verbalizing what happened, but it is a challenge. This is one reason why people may be reluctant to talk openly about their experience. It sounds odd. It's just difficult to communicate:

> I knew at the time that I could never describe it. I knew I could never fully bring it back. There were not even words to describe it. I would never ever be able to talk to other people about this because it was something I just couldn't explain.

Often people draw on metaphors in trying to describe what they experienced. One woman said:

> It's just such an overwhelming experience. It's like giving birth. You never really forget. In essence, I was giving birth to myself. I felt an energy which is still there. I think once you experience these things they almost become part of the genetic makeup of your body, so you can get back into it, like a dancer can get back into pliés. You're never the same after you've experienced it.

During a quantum change of the mystical type, people typically become aware of a nonmaterial level of reality that is difficult to put into words. For some this is a new awareness. Others had some prior belief in a nonmaterial realm of reality, but their epiphany is a direct experience of it that leaves them utterly convinced of its existence.

> It validated for me that there are more things out there than we are aware of, that we have the ability to overcome our animal nature and tap into higher realms. I remember Helen Keller came to talk to us when I was in the sixth grade, and told us about the day when

Annie Sullivan was telling her a story about God. At first Helen couldn't understand what Annie meant, but then she connected: "Wow, I always knew something was there, but I didn't know its name." This woman, who was deaf and mute, had the knowledge that something else was there, a knowledge that beyond all this there is something extraordinary, whatever name we want to put to it. I just wish that everyone could have this kind of experience.

We found that because of this ineffable quality of quantum change, our participants were often relieved to learn that others had had similar experiences.

I've tried to explain this experience to a few people, but of course, unless a person has been through it, it's impossible to understand. I was elated to read the article because it's nice to know that I'm not out here all alone.

2. Noetic Quality

Usually a mystical quantum change includes the experience of being given a message, of having an important truth revealed. This is one way in which it resembles the insightful type. The message comes into consciousness with great force and with an immediate sense of certitude. In the mystical type of quantum change there is a sense of *receiving* the message, of its being imparted from without. When an awe-inspiring presence is felt, the message is usually experienced as coming from that presence. This element of being acted upon, of having the message imparted from an Other, is not ordinarily part of the insightful type of quantum change, where the truth is experienced as happening internally or as having an unknown origin.

I was out in the desert, out in the middle of nowhere, on a Saturday afternoon. I'd just finished some practice shooting, and I wasn't doing very well. There were a few other people around. I'll never forget it, as long as I live. It was 3:30 in the afternoon. It was hot, really hot for a spring day. I can still see myself standing in that tank top and jean short-shorts. I had my long hair in a braid. There was a hot wind blowing. I was talking to this friend, and he told me that he was going back east, where he had come from. It was just something he said, and suddenly this light was there. I'm thinking

*that it's so hot and so bright out, and all of a sudden I realize,
"Good Lord, is this light inside me?" And just like that I said,
"Yeah, I guess I'm going to have to go back east, too." There it was.
He asked me, "Will you be coming back to New Mexico?" I was
still in this strange state, whatever it was, and I said, "Yeah, I'm
coming back. I think I'm going to go to school." Out of the clear
blue sky! And I had this feeling, like a brush against my cheek. It
happened when I said I would come back and go to school. The
voice inside me said, "Yes. That's it. That's it. Pack yourself up, do
what you have to do, and then come back." It kept me from divorc-
ing my husband. I came back to him, and I did go back to school.*

Sometimes the message seems to be quite specific in its instruction.
This was the beginning of a set of experiences that changed a young
man's life:

*I was in college in San Diego. I'd just finished the semester there.
My friend and I had planned to go to Mexico for the summer to
travel, but just as I was leaving college, after having finished my
last finals, some little voices started to speak to me. They said,
"Why don't you go to Los Angeles?" It was kind of bizarre. So I got
back to the apartment, and I just started to walk around, because I
was torn between following this impulse to go to Los Angeles and
going with my friend to Mexico. Anyway, I decided to kind of just
pack it up and go to Los Angeles. I put my sleeping bag in my car
and bought a six-pack and started to drive up to Los Angeles.*

*On the way this little voice said, "You know, you've been
asking a lot of questions." I was studying science at the time in
college, and I was asking my astronomy professor, "Where did we
come from?" My astronomy professor started explaining about
the big bang theory. I said that's almost as ridiculous as what religion supports. I was also taking a botany class, and I asked my
professor what makes a seed germinate. He said, "Don't worry
about it. I'm not going to put that kind of stuff on the test."*

*So I had been asking these kinds of questions. I'm on the
road to Los Angeles, and this little voice says, "You know, you've
been asking a lot of questions. You're going to find out what the
purpose of your life is." I'm driving to Los Angeles, fully aware
that what I was doing was very strange. I had my life in San
Diego. My girlfriend would be wondering where I was. My friend*

and I were supposed to go to Mexico. Yet, as I drove, I just felt like I was doing what I needed to be doing. I wound up in Redondo Beach, and I got out of my car.

I slept on the beach that night, which was very uncharacteristic of me. I wasn't the kind of guy who would generally just sleep on the beach, but I had my sleeping bag and it was a summer night. Before I went to sleep I got on my knees. Now, the only praying I'd ever done in my life was the prayers in the Catholic church, but I got on my knees and I said, "You know, God, this is really really strange for me. I don't even believe in You. As a matter of fact, I feel hostility when I see people who talk about You." And all of a sudden I just broke into tears. I began to weep, and weep, and weep, and weep, and weep. I don't know how long it went on. It may have been half an hour, or an hour. I just wept. I felt this overwhelming sense of peace and joy. Ecstasy. I had certainly experienced being intoxicated under the influence of alcohol and pot and coke and so forth, but this feeling of intoxication was just so much different. It left me feeling so peaceful, and it was very very dramatic.

When I drove back home and got together with my friends, they could tell that I had changed. I cut my hair. I stopped drinking. I wasn't interested in it anymore; stopped smoking pot and taking drugs. There was just a sort of peace and a feeling of being intoxicated that I had at that time. Of course that feeling, over the last sixteen years, comes and goes. It's not an everlasting kind of feeling. For me, it's just the nature of maintaining a religious life to develop and deepen the peace and the intoxication that I still continue to feel.

Another woman, beset with alcohol problems, had had an experience that included all of the mystical elements described earlier and that contained a message she struggled to carry with her in sobriety. She was working at home at her desk, with her children playing on the floor beside her. She was dead tired and was just thinking about stopping for a beer, when—

A voice came into my mind and said, "Everything will be all right; I am here to protect you, and I will be with you always." I can't begin to explain what I felt at that moment; I have never felt that way before. Those few simple words echoed in my head, and a blanket of warmth and love wrapped around me. As the voice was talking, I felt intensely protected and loved. For a long time I couldn't move, and I wanted it never to end.

People often speak of hearing a voice during a quantum change experience. It is more than a metaphor but less than a literal sensory experience. It is "as if" a voice were speaking, but usually there are no audible words, and others do not hear it. It is distinct from auditory hallucination, too, in that the person is completely sure that the voice is somehow internal and only "like" a voice. One woman observed:

It's not a literal voice that comes down and says, 'Take two steps to the right.' It's more like a sense of a presence of something. It's not like you're prepared for these kinds of experiences, and you never know where or when they're going to occur, but you can be open to them.

Perhaps this was Joan of Arc's experience, sometimes caricatured as hallucinations of madness. Great religious leaders such as Mahatma Gandhi (Mohandas K. Gandhi), often have a clear sense of what it is they are meant to do, directed to do, must do—again not hearing an actual voice but aware of a clarity that is "as if" a voice were speaking to them. One of our participants described it thus:

First I had these goose bumps on my face. Then I had this voice, sort of like inner talk. It's an inner voice or something inside that says "Yes." If something is wrong for me, the voice won't be there. Now, it's not like you and I speaking. It's kind of a sixth sense, and it takes away fear. I'm not afraid at these times. I don't question it. It just says to me softly—and I'm going to say "says" for lack of better words, though it's more like a feeling that pushes me, guides me—but it says softly, "Just go," or "Just do," or "Just say," or it says to be with certain people. Usually, of course, I have to make choices for myself, right or wrong, very inconsequential, but on major issues that will change my life, that voice is there. Or if I'm connected to someone and my presence or my actions will influence them, this feeling is there. Sometimes I will see—now this sounds

so airy-fairy—but sometimes I see this light, something like a
flame. It's bright around wherever it is that I'm headed for, what-
ever is the right direction. That's the best I can explain it.

3. Transiency

In mystical experience there is a particular period of awareness that
is experienced as markedly different from normal consciousness. It
may last only for a few seconds or minutes, or rarely certain altered-
state aspects of mystical experience may linger for as long as a few
days, but then there is a distinct fading of the experience. This is a
common aspect of the mystical type of quantum change: a period of
distinctly altered consciousness, followed by a fading of the acute
experience. Those with an insightful type of quantum change are
more likely to have a moment of distinct realization, a "bam," but
not one that seems a markedly altered state of consciousness. There
is a continuum here, though, and it can be difficult to classify quantum changes in the gray area.

One common aspect of altered awareness is the experience of
enhanced acuity of sensation and perception. One woman said, "I
felt a tingling. I was so charged. Things were just more *real*. Colors
were more vibrant, and smells were smellier." For some who have a
mystical experience without quantum change, the event can leave
them with a longing or hunger to reexperience it: "I did a good deal
of searching after that and really went downhill in my life. I got actually suicidal and very discouraged because I couldn't get the experience back again." Quantum changers, though, rarely voice such intense longing. Even though the mystical consciousness has faded,
they are usually left with a sense of certainty and permanence that
remains with them.

4. Passivity

In the midst of a mystical quantum change, people often feel out of
control. For a period of time, ranging from a few seconds to a few
days, they experience their mind or body responding to a will outside their own. Again, in the insightful type, there may be little or no
distinct period of altered consciousness at the outset. There is less a
sense of being temporarily suspended or out of control.

Although these brief passivity experiences can sound quite bizarre, they happen to people who show no indications of psychosis before or afterward. The "crazy" sound of these experiences is one common reason for reluctance to discuss them with others. Sometimes it is as simple as feeling physically held or restrained:

> When I was twelve, I was so depressed that I thought about committing suicide. We had gone up to Yellowstone National Park, and my dad was really hammering at me about "Isn't this beautiful? Don't you love this? Get outta the car and enjoy this. I'm doing this for your own good." I got out of the car, and we were at the "grand canyon" of Yellowstone. I went to the railing, and the rocks down below looked like pillows. It would've been nice to just step off the edge and land in those pillows. What happened was that I felt these hands grab my shoulders and a voice said to me, "Don't," and so I didn't, and I never went to the edge again during the whole trip. It was like at that time I was being protected. It didn't matter how much my father talked. It was like I had this protective shield around me and it was just bouncing off. It only lasted for a little while, but it saved my life.

Other out-of-control experiences are more elaborate:

> One day—I was thirty-five then—I was at my mother's house, sitting in the den watching some TV, and I felt a sort of pull. It felt like sometimes when you're shaken real quick by somebody and you're kind of surprised. It felt like a sudden shake. It was like there were some people and they were saying, "Come with us for a minute," only they really weren't saying that. They were just more or less beckoning. My first response was "No way," but that didn't seem to stop it. I didn't see the people like in a vision, because a vision is almost like you see something right in front of you and you can touch it. This wasn't really a vision. It was more like just in my mind. My mind could see it. It was sort of gray, not black and white and not colored, but just gray. Yet it was also like it wasn't in my head. It was off to the side a little bit. I don't know how to explain it. There were maybe three to five people, and several of them were tall. I remember them being tall—a couple of men and a couple of women, but not real distinguished. I didn't recognize any of them. The thing that was so distinguishing to me was that they were trying to comfort me and telling me that it was all right.

That was what stood out. I was curled up, sort of in a fetal position more or less, and they were trying to get me to relax and saying, "It's OK." It sounds strange, but that's the feeling I had, that I was in a fetal position, really tight and really tense, and they were try-ing to tell me, "Relax, relax," but they didn't say those words. It was just more of a feeling.

Then it was like I was sort of moved over to the side, and I could still see and hear myself there. I found I couldn't talk and I knew that I wasn't with me anymore. It was like my body was separated from me, but yet I could still see me. I was kind of standing over on the side, and I couldn't talk. For three days I walked around, and it was like everything that came out of my mouth wasn't what was like me. I could see both things. If you think of your body as just a shell run by a computer like a Star Trek *android, then it's like somebody new was at the controls. Whereas you're used to a habit of doing things a certain way, the habit is different. It's a different touch, it's a different sight, a dif-ferent sense of observation. I kept my mouth shut because I knew that things were going to come out that were different from what I did before, and there wasn't that control that I had held before, and my anger would come out.*

It wasn't frightening. I was actually very angry at the time because I wanted to be in control. I didn't want somebody else or anything else to be in control. That's probably why it was sort of dramatic, because I just don't like relinquishing control. Not that I understand what happened or what went on. It's OK, but I still wish it could have been more logical. I didn't really hear any voices or anything. It was more like they were trying to soothe me and comfort me and say, "Don't worry, just relax." It was kind of a soothing feeling, like when a mother holds a baby.

Out of context, this could easily be mistaken for a psychotic epi-sode, but it occurred within an ordinary life that was transformed dramatically for the better. The clearest change that she experienced in herself was a profound and enduring sense of peacefulness. Her prior personality had resembled the classic description of "Type A" personality[21]: tense, impatient, judgmental, chronically angry, and obsessed with being in control. In contrast, she described herself af-ter quantum change in this way: "I don't have to rush out and get the things that I want. I can wait and be relaxed in waiting, rather than anxious. I'm much more patient in solving problems, because I see that it'll happen in its own time."

5. Unity

People who have a mystical experience often have a powerful and direct experience of unity with other people, with nature, with the universe, with everything. It is as though the boundaries of individual identity drop away and the person perceives an interconnectedness of all being. In the mystical type of quantum change, this new perception seems to "stick" and stay with the person over time, rather than being a transient experience. This enduring experience of connectedness can also occur when the quantum change is primarily insightful in nature: it is the *essence* of the insight. Chapter 9 relates one woman's story in which unity was a major theme. More often, though, this experience seems to accompany the mystical type. Another woman, quoted in Chapter 3, had reached a point of desperation regarding how to parent an adolescent daughter who was leaving the house in the middle of the night. When we left her on page 26, she had just said, "Oh, dear God, help me. What can I do here? You're going to have to help me. I just can't handle this." She continued:

> *And suddenly there was a reassurance, there was just sort of a wave of knowing that everything was going to be all right and that I didn't need to worry about her anymore. All of a sudden the desperation was gone and in its place was this assurance, this peace that she was going to be all right and that I could just let go. I could surrender my concern for her and just love her. I knew that I didn't need to say anything else to her, that I didn't need to be concerned. I felt at peace. I felt reassured. I felt loved, too, like there was a union; I was a part of something that was a loving, peaceful thing, something a lot bigger than me—something loving, something caring, something that was going to take care of her, too. It was as if I was being encompassed and she would be too. She was going to be all right, going to be OK. It lasted just a minute or two, but things were different, and when it was over, the knowledge was still there. The feeling was gone but the certainty was still there. There was a relaxation, and I quit crying. There wasn't anything to cry about anymore. I remember I got up and went into the bath-*

room, and when I came out I went to bed and went to sleep. I don't know what time she came in, but it didn't matter then. It was as if a big load had been lifted off me. I didn't have to worry about this child anymore. I was very surprised. It was not what I expected at all.

Sometimes the experience is one of merging with a particular person or object:

It was not like a lightning bolt to the head, but it certainly struck me. I was watching an educational special about a volcano. The more I saw this volcano move and change and grow, the lava flowing forth and the redness and the hotness of it, the more I felt in tune with that volcano and more and more a part of it. I had this sensation of no distance between me and this mechanical device and the volcano, like we were truly all part of one thing. I became aware that there is so much out there that we aren't aware of. This volcano represented to me the amount and the intensity of change that occurs in our planet and in ourselves. I felt the reality of so many levels of existence, of being able to tap into it. I kept a diary, and I remember writing that I had heard the voice again. It's not a literal voice that comes down and says something like "Take two steps to the right." It's more like a sense of a presence of something. It's not like you're prepared for these kinds of experiences, and you never know where or when they're going to occur, but you can be open to them. It was the lava. It was just a eureka kind of thing. I saw the lava and the sparks, and the fire just catapulted me into the sky. The experience was like a little volcano. The actual boom happened when I saw the sparks, and I said, "Wow, do that again!"

Maslow described it this way[22]:

The whole of the world is seen as unity, as a single rich live entity. In other of the peak experiences, . . . one small part of the world is perceived as if it were for the moment all of the world.

6. Transcendence

One of the more profound unity experiences that we heard emerged from a moment of dreadful suffering. It is a story that also illustrates mystical transcendence of physical limitations. A young woman had gone to Mexico for an abortion at a time when they were illegal in the United States. This is part of her story:

I was lying on the table with the horrible stirrups. The experience was so painful. It was unbelievable. I could hear screaming in my ears, and I saw stars. I literally saw stars, like in the comic books when somebody is hit on the head. Everything was swirling. I had never experienced pain like this. It was beyond description. It was so bad that all of a sudden I had left my body. Let me tell you, when you leave your body, you know it. You just know. I mean, you're not in your body anymore. I didn't see or hear what was going on in the room. I had left it behind, and my consciousness was soaring through the universe. I was going at the speed of light—that's the only way I can describe it. It was so fast. I was speeding past all these stars and galaxies. It was not a pleasant experience. I was so dizzy, and I was going so fast. It was scary, terrifying, and yet it was very beautiful. It's really hard to describe because it was the most horrible and most wonderful thing you could experience. I guess all the contradictions are there.

What I saw in that experience I can't totally describe. I knew at the time that I saw all of creation. I saw heaven, and I saw hell. When I saw hell, it wasn't anything like what the preachers would tell you. It was more like all the suffering gathered together. We didn't believe in hell when I was growing up. I was Episcopalian, and I guess most Episcopalians don't concentrate at all on hell. I saw everything anybody has ever thought of. I knew that absolutely everything anybody had ever thought of was real, that anything we had ever conceived of somehow existed. All of creation was so vast, and you could see it in this split second of time. All of creation, you might say then, would be mind. It's what I saw. I also knew that there is much more than the physical body and that when you die you go on. I saw that in that experience.

And then I just felt so at peace. It was very, very, very calming, because I knew something really important. I knew I was no longer limited by the physical. I think the pain was so extreme that it forced my consciousness out of my body. I was able to transcend the physical, to see beyond the physical limitations. I have never feared death since then, nor have I ever experienced depression, which was a major change for me.

7. Awe

One common characteristic that distinguishes mystical from insightful quantum changes is the experience of being in the presence of an
Other, of something outside of and greater than oneself. This experience has been described as awe and is often difficult to express in
words. This is what happened to a desperate woman contemplating
a murder–suicide, whose story began in Chapter 3:

> *That night I remembered that I had a religion once. I am not a
> church member, not a religious person. I'm a spiritual person, but I
> had no affiliation to any religion, so this is not going to be one of
> these born-again Christian stories. I'm not going to tell you that I
> suddenly saw the light. But I did have this Christian background,
> and that winter night I suddenly remembered some of the things
> that I had read. So that night I asked for help. It was about two or
> three in the morning. I said, "Please, help me!" From the bottom of
> my heart, I asked for help. I said, "Please, show me what you want
> me to do." Suddenly it was like this angel appeared in my mind,
> and this voice said to me, "Turn to me." Just like that. I felt a pres-
> ence. I didn't really see a vision. There was just a feeling of light. I
> opened my heart, and something came in. Whether it was from me
> going out or it was coming in I can't say. It was the meaning that
> was important. It wasn't a long, drawn-out thing. It wasn't leading
> up to anything in that sense, and it wasn't from anybody else. It
> wasn't my mother or anybody else I knew. There was nothing else
> in that experience except that it was like I had finally turned to the
> divine. I didn't see a blinding flash or anything else, but somehow I
> just knew everything from then on was going to be all right. It was
> like I suddenly burst through and let go, and everything, everything
> just changed. There was help right there, right there. The whole
> thing lasted maybe thirty minutes or so, and then I fell asleep. I re-
> member relaxing and being able to fall asleep. I'm foggy about how
> long it took, but I know that it was in the middle of the night and it
> was close to dawn when I finally fell asleep. It was the most amaz-
> ing night of my life.*

A mother described this encounter, which had occurred more than
twenty years earlier:

When I was seventeen, I had a religious experience. I was really, really into religion and the Bible then. We were on a camping trip, and that night in the tent I couldn't go to sleep. Everybody else was sleeping. Suddenly the tent filled up with this pink light, and this figure came and stood before me. Now, I thought it was a figure of Jesus. Another person might have seen something else, but to me it was a figure of Jesus, and the words were "Why do you doubt my words?" The next morning I woke up. I picked up my Bible, and I could understand what I was reading. It changed my ability to read and understand.

This sense of awe, of being in a presence, often (but not always) overlaps with the experience of unity described above. The examples of unity experiences given earlier also contain this component of awe.

8. Positivity

When a mystical quantum changer feels the presence of another being, almost always he or she experiences the nature of that presence as profoundly loving. Again, the experience of being cared for is often difficult to explain because it is unlike anything previously experienced:

On December 25, 1981, I was driving home from work—Christmas Day. It was approximately 7:30 or 8:00 in the morning. It was a beautiful clear day. The sky was very blue. It was a cold day—sharp, crisp. I was in my car. I was driving east on I-40, and all of a sudden I knew it. It just happened. I mean it was just "Bam!" There it was. I can't explain it to you in adequate words. I felt incredible warmth. I felt that there was a presence in the car with me. I felt incredible acceptance, love, a sense of well-being, euphoria, everything's going to be well. I choose to believe, and I chose to believe at that time, that the presence that was in the car was Jesus Christ. I didn't see him. This was not a visual experience. What I felt was incredible warmth, an incredible sense of well-being. I felt loved like I had never been loved in my life.

In Raymond Moody's book, Life After Life, *the people who had died briefly talk about moving toward this light and feeling*

*an incredible love that they had never felt before in their lives—
so much so that if they had been given the choice of going on toward the light or coming back, they all wanted to go on toward
that light. I think what I felt was just a fraction of that. Well, I
don't know if this is true or not, but, I just don't think it was all
the love that God has to give. I felt that it was just a fraction of
it. I felt nonjudgmental love. I felt total acceptance for whoever I
was. In a spiritual sense, I knew that I was not alone, that there
was a purpose for the universe, that I was going to be OK. It was
so overpowering, so overwhelming, that I'm going down the free-
way and I'm crying and I'm grinning from ear to ear. Never in
my life, never, have I had a feeling like that in my life, never,
never.*

*I read that God speaks to us in quiet moments. Well, this
was one of those moments. God was saying, "Look, I love you.
I know it's hard and you don't understand, and I'm thanking you
for not shaking your fist at me and cursing me out and taking
that route. You've got the right approach. Thank you for letting
me in."*

The following was the turning point for a physician who had struggled long with drug addiction:

*I was lying there saying this prayer. With every breath I'd say, with
all sincerity in my heart, "God, please help me to trust you." I realized, "I'm miserable. There is nothing I can do except turn to God. I
can't call my girlfriend, because she's not there. I can't call counselors or sponsors. None of that's going to help. So with every breath
for about five minutes I kept saying, "Dear God, please help me to
trust you." And then I had this new thought, which was not my
own thought, to say this prayer: "Oh, God, please bathe me in the
light of your love."*

*Whew! All of a sudden, for about two or three seconds, I had
this thing happen to me that was just out of this world. I mean it
was like warm and wonderful and unmistakable, and like nothing that had ever happened to me in my life. I just got this
warm, wonderful, beautiful feeling. I can't even try in words to
describe what it was like. When you take intravenous morphine,
you get this sudden euphoric thing. That's similar to what happened, but drugs pale in comparison to what this felt like. It was*

really unique. That was the first time I knew something was really going on. I didn't want it to stop. I wanted to keep it happening.

9. Distinctiveness

Finally, there is no question that the mystical experience is distinctively different from ordinarily experienced reality. A number of people described their experience as a "boom" in which their awareness suddenly shifted to reveal a new plane or truth. Consciousness is temporarily altered in a mystical experience, and in the mystical type of quantum change it leaves behind a permanent shift in perception as well.

One example is a frequent element in mystical quantum change experiences that is usually called "light," although it is unlike ordinary light. Often it doesn't seem to come from anywhere in particular and it is not visible to others present. Several of those who told us their stories said that it was as though the light was not *falling upon* them but rather was *emanating from* them. Light is referred to in several stories already quoted in this chapter. Here is another in which light was particularly central:

It started with the birth of my son, which was a completely spiritual experience for me. It was a natural birth, which back then wasn't popular. Something happened. There was just a shift. My body was trembling, and I was moved and I was crying. By the time I got to the hospital I was in hard labor, and then they asked me if I could wait because the delivery room was full and didn't I want something for the pain. I remember looking at the doctor and saying "What pain? There isn't any pain. This doesn't hurt." I can remember it just being exhilarating, like my whole body was vibrating. It was exhilarating. It was almost like an orgasm—something like that. "Pain? What are you talking about? This is ecstatic!" It was like the opposite of pain, really. My body was streaming with energy.

The doctor who was delivering my baby was someone who didn't normally use natural childbirth, but he saw how important it was to me. We were very much connected on a real intimate level, the doctor and I, there in the birthing room. It happened in just a moment of time. We kind of entered another way of being with each other. He delivered the baby, and then I started crying. I was emotionally touched, you know, that kind of crying where it isn't crying. It's kind of exuding out of you. Your face is sheeted with tears. That kind of crying. And there was a light. There was light everywhere. All I know is it was like awe—awful awesome—wonder. It was as if I were joined with some mystery, and that was the most important piece of it. That is actually my experience now, but I'm getting ahead of the story. I was so grateful. It was such a miracle. It was a shocking miracle. The doctor felt it too, and the nurse who was there in the room, and an attendant who was there in the room who had breathed with me.

It was as if there were light in the room. Then they put the baby on me, and the doctor asked me if I was OK. I said that I was, thanks. I hadn't been a religious person at all, not at all. I had really turned my back on spirituality or God or religion or anything like that. Then the doctor started to cry and said he was struck by the miracle of all of it, too. Now this is a guy who delivered babies all the time in the hospital. There were people lined up in the halls waiting for the room, to have babies. There was just something really unique about this birth for everybody who was in the room. I know he remembers it. Then it continued when they put me in another room and wrapped me in this warm towel. The light continued there. It was like the light was coming out from me, like I was the center of it and it was just coming out from me, and my body was streaming out.

When they brought my baby to me in the middle of the night, it was magical. He wouldn't eat; you know how babies won't suckle right away. I didn't know that, so I thought maybe something was wrong. I thought, "Should I unwrap him?" No, I was afraid to unwrap him, so I just had him be on my chest all bundled up and I talked to him, but it wasn't out-loud talking. I told him what kind of mother I was going to be. I promised him that I wouldn't hold on to him like an object, that I would let him be of the world, and it was as if God were present. It was as if that talk was being witnessed by God.

In many aspects of their experience, and on all the personal characteristics we measured (such as age, gender, and personality type), there were no significant differences between those who had insightful versus mystical quantum changes. Yet there were some differences. Those with mystical epiphanies were twice as likely to remember the exact time of day it occurred, even though the insightful quantum changes had occurred much more recently on average (two and a half years versus fourteen years ago). Since these are people who contacted us to tell their stories, perhaps the mystical type of change leaves a more salient memory that even decades later is still clearly identifiable as something out of the ordinary, a distinct turning point. Those who had the epiphany type of quantum change were twice as likely to say that they had felt completely loved, that they had a "vision," and that they felt themselves to be in the hands of a Higher Power during the event. They were four times more likely to report "hearing" a voice and five times more likely to say that someone had been praying for them at the time of their quantum change. They were also more likely to use God language in talking about their experience.

The five chapters that follow present a fascinating array of epiphanies. The first of them, Chapter 11, is a unique firsthand account of the mystical elements described above. Its uniqueness derives from the fact that on the day the epiphany happened, this man was driving his car and had a tape recorder with him, making a voice letter to the first author and his wife. It may be the only tape-recorded account of its kind. Consequently, a moment after it occurred the driver was able to describe his experience as it unfolded, and fortunately he asked us to save the tape. It provides an unusually fresh and immediate description, whereas most such accounts are recollections at some distance from the event. Such recollections are often colored by the subsequent consolidation process, in which the person seeks to understand and integrate the event. To provide this contrast of perspectives, Chapter 11 contains both a direct transcription of the event just as it happened and the man's reflections on it now, after having two decades in which to integrate it.

The story that is told in Chapter 12, "Something Like a Star," contains all nine of the elements described above as characteristic of the mystical type of quantum change. It is a particularly clear illustration of *passivity* in epiphanies—of feeling in the presence and temporarily under the control of that which is much greater than oneself. Another man was startled to hear "A Voice in the Fireplace" (Chapter 13) that transformed him from a tense and tightly controlled person to one who is serene and comfortable with his newfound intuition.

Some quantum changes occur as "born-again" Christian experiences, and Chapter 14 is one of these. Often the term "born again" is associated with a conversion from no religion to a fervent Christian faith. In this case, the recipient was a lifelong practicing Catholic whose faith and being were profoundly deepened by a sudden, unexpected encounter. Although some might assert that born-again experiences are qualitatively distinct, the similarities of this story to other mystical quantum changes are clear. Most of the nine elements are again evident.

The storyteller of "Trampoline" (Chapter 15), by contrast, had already experienced a Christian conversion some years before, which he describes as being "totally different" from the quantum change that occurred instantaneously at the moment of his traumatic injury. Certainly his preexisting religious faith provided a framework within which to understand and describe what happened to him. Yet his quantum change provided an unexpected and transforming twist to what anyone would expect to be a devastating tragedy.

11

THE RELUCTANT MYSTIC

Authors' note: *He was driving across the plains of eastern Oregon in 1980. Beside him on the seat of his car was an inexpensive tape recorder, and to pass the time he was recording a letter to friends. He chatted about bumper stickers, using old chimney bricks for remodeling, the hay in the fields, and an album he was recording. Behind his voice were the roar of the engine and the drone of traffic. He finished the first side of the tape just as he pulled off the road at Boardman to have supper. On the second side of the tape, his voice had a strikingly different sound: breathless, shaken, struggling to find adequate words. What follows is a transcription of the immediate experience as told in his own words at the time.*

*   *   *

I'm back on the road again, and since I talked to you last an amazing thing has happened to me. It is totally positive, and I'm so glad I have this tape recorder to be able to talk with you about it. I just had supper and was just getting back on the road. Oh! I've been crying a lot because something joyful happened and, God, it's just been sort of all bubbling out of me. I've been talking to myself and trying to get it all in perspective, so pardon my breathlessness and however it pours out.

93

I guess I've just had the kind of experience that Saul must have had on the road to Damascus. That's the closest experience that I can relate this to. I'm out of breath. I've just had such an experience of God! I was driving along, just coming through all of that mostly boring country that I was talking to you about on the other side of the tape, and there was nothing in particular spectacular happening. In fact, I was really just kind of bored, driving along. It's real boring, dusty country. All of a sudden, out of just absolutely nowhere—I mean no spectacular clouds, no beautiful mountains, no pretty ocean, no sunset or anything—just out of God-literally-knows-where, I just got a sweeping experience of the presence of the *Holy Spirit*, I guess. That sounds kind of strange coming from me, because I don't talk like this very often, but I was just moving along and, whammo, I went all goose bumps and all the hairs on my arms and legs just started standing on end, and I was just kind of full of electricity. Not exactly a voice or anything like that, but kind of a bright, shining message came through to me that said . . . it was just sort of saying yes—a very, very big important yes, followed by a sort of thought outside of myself that came through in the words . . . the best that I can come up with is "Yes, you do understand me, and here is some more understanding," which is just . . . I'm starting to cry again . . . which is just an amazingly joyful experience for me. Here I am riding along by myself, and all of a sudden this message comes to me and I feel happy and fulfilled, and I feel on course, driving along this stupid, barren road.

I guess what that all comes from is a kind of unasked question that I've had, or an unverbalized question anyway—I know God's been hearing it—about "Am I interpreting you right, God, as I do my workshops and music?" Of course, what that's all talking about is God. Sometimes just because of being in schools it's not politically right to be saying "This is God that I'm talking about folks!"—but of course that's what I'm trying to bring to people.

I guess the question that I've been having on and off through all the years, and probably will have again, though certainly not as much after this experience, is "Am I right? Am I interpreting you right? Is this valid?" I feel it's valid, and that's what I'm staking my life on, and my thoughts say it's valid, and my emotions say it's valid, but somehow or other I guess I've needed some kind of sign. I get those signs in validations from my friends and from concerts. People react to my songs and my workshops and say that they're good, and that's been very important to me, but, wow—to just be driving along a road, with my mind kind of blank, just driving along, and all of a sudden for the validation to come *then*, to come from God outside of myself when I wasn't looking for it! After a concert I would be expecting somebody to validate me, or after a workshop I would be expecting that, but for that kind of intense spiritual validation to just sweep over me, just out of the blue—in fact, not even out of the blue, but out of the dust of driving along the road—has just blown me away and has done an awful lot to remove some of those fringy doubts, my question about, well, is this just an intellectual thing that I'm going through? Is it just rational? Is it just that kind of experience?

Sometimes, about five percent of the time, I think, "Is this whole thing really, really God? Am I really helping that come through to folks?" And "YES! YES! That's right!" God just said that to me! And it was almost as if, it was almost as if a lonely misunderstood person had come to me and said, "Thank you for understanding, thank you for listening to me." I'm starting to really realize, in what I'm feeling right now, that God is just as lonely as any of us are, and God needs somebody to listen, and God needs company, too. God is thankful that there are some people who are trying to explore what the depths of God are about and not accepting God or taking God in some kind of superficial way in order to take care of needs for power or something like that.

Anyway, that's kind of what I've been going through. And an amazing thing happened right after that experience that obviously I'm still partly going through. Right after that experience I looked back at that same landscape that moments before I had been thinking, "This is just really boring."

[*The voice stops. When it returns, the roar of the engine is gone.*]

I decided to pull off. I can't concentrate. I'm going all funny while I'm trying to drive, and the tape machine keeps clicking off, which is the reason for all these pauses and starts and stops. Anyway, all that stuff that had seemed really really boring . . . all of a sudden everything was really beautiful. Everything! I mean, I looked out and said, "God, look at that! This is the *earth*, and all of that dust out there is really beautiful, and all of that *nothing* is just so beautiful and so full," and I became so aware again that God is all around us—everywhere, of course.

Words are so weak to explain that. And it occurred to me, "How can we be involved in a search for something that's already here?" We operate inside of this funny little human mind that we have, that is too small to comprehend that God is so large and so all pervasive and so close that we can't even see God. God is *us*—God is outside of us and inside of us and through us, all around. It's just amazing to me that God is beyond concept, and it occurs to me that in the middle of our struggle for concepts for explaining God, the concepts are useless. The reason we need to have concepts to talk about and to argue about is simply because we're just incapable of understanding things any other way, so we invent all these ways to help our finiteness so that we can have a few nails to hang our hat on. And it occurred to me, I realized that the main search is not our search for God—because God is already here with us always—that the main search is not our search for God but God's search for us. For whatever reason there is, God slipped down and jumped into me during those few moments and opened me up to all of that. I'm glad that I have you here, even if it's on this tape, to talk to because of course that brings you here. I'm thinking of you and the people I'll be trying to explain this whole thing to later on tonight, because we've shared so much together.

It occurs to me that we just really need to be in places where God can find us. I started thinking about how God is so pervasive that He finds people—that God, Spirit, He, She—finds people. . . . And it occurs to me that God speaks to people in the space that they are in, and God speaks to people from their need. I started thinking about a fellow in the workshop that I was doing in a junior high school today. We were talking about dreams and what we thought we ought to be doing in life, which is another way of talking about what God wants us to do. He said, "I used to have this dream about being a rock and roll star until I was going through the *National Geographic* one day, and I saw the pictures of all the dolphins that were being slaughtered by fishermen, and I decided, what's being a rock and roll star compared to those beautiful animals being killed? I decided I wanted to be part of stopping those animals from being killed." For whatever reason, God found that young fellow in the pages of *National Geographic* and not in the pages of Revelation. Other people God finds in the pages of Revelation because that's where they happen to be.

I'm so exhausted from this experience! But I want to keep talking.

God finds us. And the thing that is so exciting to me is that now—because of this experience that came to me, outside of me, when I wasn't looking for it—I'm really able to say not that I'm right (that's not the point, not in terms of right and wrong) but at least that I am now sure that the way that I have chosen or have been led into is right; it's valid. God has said yes to that, and there's just no doubt in my mind.

That doesn't mean that that way is right for everybody. The excitingness of this is "Yes, that is *a right way.*" That it is possible for God to give that kind of spiritual experience in the same way that I experienced it, and perhaps as powerfully, to somebody else who has another way, and that can be right, too. *Of course!* And that my work is to understand that *that's* true, and part of my work is also now to share with people this experience that I've had that shows that this way is also true. The exciting part of it is that I can honestly say that I've had an important experience of God coming to me, and the most exciting part of it is that message coming through to me when I wasn't looking for it. It wasn't a matter of standing outside under the night sky and saying "God, send me a sign that you're there." If you stand and look at the sky long enough on any given night you'll see a shooting star. I'm not saying that *couldn't* be God doing that for the person who was looking for a sign. But there certainly can be the suspicion that if a person wants a sign that what he thinks is true, and he puts himself in that particular place where he will probably get some kind of experience from nature, then he can use that to say, "Well, see, God spoke to me." The exciting part of this was that there was no way in the world I was even prepared for this, that it was an answer to a question that I've been struggling with for a long time in my life, and when I wasn't seeking the answer or seeking a sign or seeking the Presence, the Presence came through. That voice outside of me said, "Yes, you understand," and after that I had the feeling that "Yes you understand, and *keep going. Keep doing what you're doing, and don't give up. And please remember this moment if there are times when you do feel like giving up.*"

I know that as long as I ask for the love that I need from people I will get it, and that that's another way that God loves me. We have to understand what that phrase "Knock and it shall be opened unto you" means, really, in our lives. Asking people to love us and help us with our lives is part of what that means. That's not a new thought for me, but it certainly takes on a new dimension for me now.

Well, I'm tired. I'm glad I could share this with you while it is happening to me. I have a feeling right now of not only exhaustion—a very healthy, joyful exhaustion—but also a feeling that everything is all right. Everything is going to work, no matter in what ways or in what forms, things are going to work for us as long as we stand with the truth that we know, that God has given to us. Our relationships will work the way they're supposed to if we work at them. There is so much pain involved in our journeys, but after all it will be all right. We just have to love each other and love ourselves and ask for what we need. Everything is as it should be if we will just see it that way, and change is as it should be, and that's part of it. It doesn't mean that things should stay as they are, but the process is as it should be, because that process is God, too. Everything is God. Our pain is God, and our dissatisfaction is God, and our frustration is just God talking to us, and when we stay stuck there is a reason for staying stuck, even if it's to make us feel how bad that is so that eventually we'll move, and that's true for all of us.

The process is God's process. We really all *are* God's children, and God will take care of us and help us take care of ourselves. Friends are God's wonderful gift, and that's a way God helps us out, a practical way, through our love.

I realize that over the next few years I'm going to have to do a whole lot more sharing, like I'm doing with you now, with lots and lots of other people, to try to talk to them the way I'm talking to you and try to remember how important this has been. When you get this tape, I think it's going to be important for you to hold on to it, because I think I'll want to play this back to myself in times when I forget.

I can't think of anything else that needs saying. [*A pause; the tape stops and then starts again.*] You know me better than that. There is one more thing I need to say. I love you.

REFLECTIONS OF A RELUCTANT MYSTIC

Don Eaton[23]

I had a mystical experience in 1980 and didn't talk about it for more than 15 years. I had been on tour for two weeks in eastern Oregon, doing concerts and workshops in schools and wondering if I had just been beating my head against the wall or whether some of the messages got through. I was driving near Boardman, and I just wanted to be home, but I knew I still had a long drive ahead of me. It was hot, and I was tired. As I looked at the landscape, it was all dry dirt and rocks, and I thought to myself, "This is just really ugly, boring terrain."

All of a sudden, out of nowhere, this wave of spiritual electricity washed over me. My body and the car and the landscape and everything started turning into smaller and smaller and smaller pieces, and everything started disappearing, including myself. I didn't know if I was having a heart attack or what was happening. During those moments everything, including myself and the car and the landscape, just turned into little dots of light. A visual metaphor that captures something of what it looked and felt like is the transporter in *Star Trek*, where the person being beamed up is turned into little dots of light and goes somewhere—or nowhere. It was awesome, and it was terrifying, and it was peaceful.

I pulled the car off what was left of the highway, and what happened in the next few minutes changed my life. It was the annihilation of the self, which I had never heard or read about but now was experiencing. What I felt was the actual *experience*—not the thought, not a discussion about, but the actual experience—of being one with everything else and with God. I felt myself dissolve into it and it dissolve into me. There was no separation. There is a Japanese character for this experience which translates roughly as "This and that—no difference," or "I and Thou—the same." It was the most beautiful, awesome experience I have ever had. I have heard this described as the "drop in the ocean experience," where the ocean is God and we feel like a drop in that ocean. It *was* that experience, but what amazed and astounded me was the experience of feeling the ocean in the drop, God in me, the actual experience of unity. We are one with each other and with God and with everything. I disappeared into that space, and when I was in that moment of unity, I experienced what God is, which is absolute unconditional love and unity with everything and everyone, especially *you*. I can't find the words to tell you the ecstasy and the peace of those moments. I can't tell you the loneliness that I have lived with since coming back from that experience, yet also the joy, because even though I don't experience it all the time, I know what truth is. I know that you and I are the same. Reality is mainly space filled with thought and with love.

So there I was, at one with God, and the message that needs to be shared is the same message that came from the thirteenth-century mystics. One of them observed that the reason we can't dwell for very long in that space is that if we remained there long, the experience of the love of God would annihilate us with joy. That's what I experienced. I experienced no ego, no sense of self. That's a very old experience. You don't find mystics getting together and arguing with each other. One mystic speaks, and the others smile in recognition. There is no dogma, no drive to convert people to a particular understanding of the truth.

In that moment I suddenly *knew* some spiritual truths. I was very reluctant to talk about these in particular, because it sounds like ego, but there were some very clear messages that came through in those moments. The main one is the absolutely unconditional nature of God's love and that God's presence is in us, through us, and all around us. For me, the truths that I experienced are that there is absolutely no death, no hell, no judgment from God, no such thing as time (although we have the illusion of it). There is no such thing as space. There is a sense in which God is grateful for our search, and yet the search isn't really needed. The eye with which we look for God is the same eye with which God is looking for us. There was all of this, and more, all in that one moment.

I was not at all prepared for the experience. The next day, in fact, some voice inside me whispered, "It never happened." I felt as if the experience had never happened, and yet there was the tape I had sent. I was not brought up in a tradition that honored mysticism, and I was very skeptical of the TV evangelist version of "God spoke to me." I didn't talk about my experience until more than fifteen years after it happened. I thought that if I talked about it, I could ruin whatever positive reputation I had established. I was afraid of what people would think of me. Maybe they would think I had gone over the edge or had been converted to some New Age religion. So I just kept it to myself. What a strange thing—that we keep the most transforming experiences of our lives to ourselves because we are afraid of what people will think.

Coming back into ordinary reality, into this world, when it all started chunking back together, was one of the most difficult experiences of my life. I had been exactly where I wanted to be. I had been at peace. I had no fear. I was totally a part of God. I watched the car reassemble and myself reassemble, and I could start to see things again. I felt a wave of sadness, a physical heaviness like being made of lead, a sense of "Oh, no, I don't want to go back in there." I could feel myself already beginning to forget the experience.

As I came into focus, I looked back at that boring landscape, the rocks and the dirt and the sand, and all of it was just glowing with the presence of God. I got out of the car, and I knelt down in the earth and picked up some sand and rocks, and I experienced God in the earth. I didn't know whether I was holding it or it was holding me. It was an experience of ecstasy, which literally means "being out of your skin." Then when I got back in the car, back on the road, I picked up the tape recorder I had been using and started talking.

Coming back into ordinary reality left me with a sense of yearning that feels like pain, and the release from that is to realize that it is the yearning *itself* that is the experience of God. It is lonely to walk around in the world *knowing* that we are really all one and yet not being able to access that on demand. Ever since that time, I have wanted to go back to that place. It has to do, I think, with putting ourselves in places where we can be found, where we can rediscover that unity.

I believe that we are all mystics and that we need to tell our stories and hear each others' stories. When I tell my story to an audience of twenty people now, four of them will come up to me afterward and say that they have had such experiences in their lives that they have not shared with people because folks would think that they are crazy. A friend of mine described my experience to a psychiatrist, who kindly observed, "Obviously he was having a psychotic break and should be institutionalized." Another of my own sources of reluctance was the feeling-left-out response of some who say, "But I haven't had a mystical experience. What's wrong with me?" The point isn't whether or not we have had some dramatic experience. Usually we experience God in small epiphanies. The importance of mystical experiences isn't *who* has had them and who has not but rather *that they happen*. There are messages, I think, that are trying to get through to us to help enlighten this reality.

12

SOMETHING LIKE A STAR

My life was going to hell.

Because of my family history, I was grandiose in my financial ambitions. I got overextended into real estate just when one should not have done that in the local market.

I never got any deep satisfaction out of my job or my profession. I'm a scientist. I've always had a broad interest in science. My mother's messages kept running in my head: "Well, it's nice that you have a PhD, but you'd better still make a lot of money, and you'd better be the boss over a whole bunch of people." And so I was, and I was doing it, of course, for my parents.

Emotionally I was withdrawn from my family and from my wife. I had been very much out of touch with my feelings for most of my adult life. I was living merely in my head and my intellect. I retreated into my intellect from anything that was emotionally painful. I had given total responsibility for raising my kids to my wife.

My parents had died several years earlier, and I was using alcohol daily. Every night I'd go home and I'd start drinking, and by the end of the evening I would have consumed typically five, six, seven, eight drinks. Before I started to come unglued, I went to a John Bradshaw lecture after seeing his show on public television (PBS). That was the first time in my life I really, all of a sudden, realized that I come from a highly dysfunctional family. I started going to Adult

Children of Alcoholics meetings. My parents weren't alcoholic, but what I thought I had in common with those people was that I came from a dysfunctional family.

Yet I was still abusing alcohol. Every night I was numbing myself with alcohol, and every day I was just a workaholic at work—just frantically getting through the day, keeping busy constantly, trying to control my investments, trying to control my work.

Then I got this grandiose scheme that I was going to make hundreds of thousands of dollars by subdividing some land that I had really bought for our personal use. Of course, it was necessary to strike water on the land, so I studied all the geology and talked to the U.S. Geological Service geologist. I figured there was water under there, and we drilled a 600-foot well for a cost of six thousand dollars. It was bone dry.

That failure on top of everything else provoked more anxiety, increased my use of alcohol, and by the spring of that year I'd decided I'd better do some work with a therapist. So I went to a therapist, and when I told him about my pattern of drinking he wondered if I was an alcoholic and he suggested that I think about that. He gave me a book on alcoholic families, which actually was an unfair thing to do. What was described in the book was how the children of alcoholics are the hero, the scapegoat, and the lost child. What I saw in that was my own children. This was an incredible blow for me because I saw how I was hurting my children. Anyway, he suggested that I go to a few AA meetings to see if I fit. So I stopped drinking and I went to some AA meetings. I decided I didn't fit after a few of those, because the stories of the people who shared in those meetings didn't fit me. I had no loss of control. I drank because I wanted to, because I was in pain, and not because I couldn't stop.

A few days after I stopped drinking, all of these incredible feelings were with me, about being a failure financially, about hurting my children, about life being absolutely no fun anymore. I just felt like there was no reason to live. I'd had those feelings all my adult life, and I kept running from one thing to another looking for satisfaction in life. I flew airplanes, I played intense sports, spent a few summers overseas. I did everything that I could think of. I mean, you name it, I've tried it. Sky diving! But there was nothing, nothing that was satisfying. The new thing would produce excitement, but it would last only a little while.

So anyway, four days after I stopped drinking, I felt like I couldn't go back and drink because I'd admitted I overused it, but at the same time I was so miserable and I didn't want to live the way I was. That's when I had the first of several experiences. This was not the big one, just the prelude. I went home for lunch. I was driving back to work. I felt absolutely miserable. I felt just incredible pain, and I said, "God I don't know if you exist or not, but if you don't, I'm dead. I have nowhere else to turn. I have nothing else I can try. I've tried to do it all. I've tried to hold it together, and I just can't do it. So if you're there, please give me a sign. Something. Just to let me know that you exist." I was driving on Central Avenue between Tramway and Juan Tabo. It was a beautiful day, puffy white clouds in the sky. I was just looking up there in incredible pain, and I heard a little voice in my head, and it said, "I'm here, son." Tears came to my eyes. I felt this incredible release of all that pain, and I was stunned. I thought, "Am I hallucinating? Was this real?" I was sort of in shock. I wasn't sure if that really happened.

I got back to work: "Better think about it later, get back into doing something." I told my wife about it two days later, and I was just completely relaxed after that. By then I was convinced it was real, and I just thought, "This changes everything, all of my presumptions about life and everything else. This is incredible. God exists! There's something there. I mean, I call it God, but, you know, it's not an old man with a beard. There's something there that I wasn't aware of before in my life. My wife noticed the change. My counselor noticed the change. For the next week and a half or so, I was just sort of floating around being serene, not taking seriously anything that used to drive me up the wall, that I used to see as life and death, like money and job. I was just feeling like "This is really great. The whole ball game just changed. All the rules just changed, just because of this one little thing. Well, if God does exist, then all of this stuff that I've been spending my life worrying about is unimportant. I've been killing myself over all this, and it's not even important. There's a whole new side of life to explore, to learn about." I was just very relaxed and serene.

Meanwhile, I'm going about my work for about another week and I go back to one of these AA meetings again, and I become convinced that I'm not an alcoholic. So I told my counselor, "OK, I tried it. I'm not an alcoholic, but why is it that I have these kids who just sound like they come from an alcoholic family?" I know now that that can happen in any dysfunctional family. Anyhow, I did stop drinking. I took a look at it, I considered it anyway, and I realized that drinking was just a pattern, and I had to break it. It was ridiculous to feel like I needed to anesthetize myself every evening.

Now in the meantime, my counselor gets in cahoots with my wife and tells her, "I don't think this is going to last because he's already decided he's not really an alcoholic. I think treatment would be a good idea." I think it's unethical what he did, but he gets together this confrontation, an intervention where you get the wife and everyone else together, and he's saying, "Why don't you consider going to treatment?" They were expecting a big fight, a protest, objections, but I was still feeling very serene, and so I just said, "OK, I'll take it. This will be fun. This will be a new experience. This will be something interesting. Maybe I'll learn something about myself." And so I went to treatment.

Now one thing that they did, and there is a lot of talk about whether this is sound or not, is what they call "survivors' week." It's the second week of the program. They first teach you what abuse is, and coming from my family, the stuff I thought was normal, now I know was highly abusive. The second thing is that they get you into guided imagery and they take you back in time, back to when the abuse happened. You recall the abuse, and it's a very powerful technique. I saw somebody just end up curled up on the floor because they recalled something that happened to them when they were two or three years old. I was only in my first week, and one of the people in our group was talking about her sexual abuse experience with her father, and already I knew I was one of the survivors, too. I already knew consciously that I had been sexually abused. I was fourteen years old, and that was my deepest, deepest, darkest secret. I told my wife that this guy molested me, but I had never told anyone how long the abuse went on, how many times, or the details of exactly what happened. This guy was a fifty-year-old pedophile who ran a club where I was a member. I must have had "victim" written all over me, "needy child" written all over me, and he took advantage of that. I felt so much shame from what happened that I just couldn't talk about it back then. I couldn't share it with anyone. I knew they were going to get to that in my treatment the next week, and I was really scared.

I think, in a program like that you actually benefit more from the other patients than from the therapists' advice. Just knowing that you're all in this together and you're not alone is wonderful. Anyhow, I had this sense that "Well, it's nice to know that God is out there somewhere, like maybe up in the sky," but I heard a lot of people there talking about the necessity of feeling some spirit within you. So, on Saturday afternoon, facing the beginning of this survivors' week on Monday, I went to my room to read one of the books they gave us. I'm lying on my bed thinking about this, and feeling very uncomfortable because I didn't want to face it. I had seen a little of the guided imagery stuff, and I thought, "Maybe I could just sort of pretend to take a little bit of God and put it within me," because that first week, when I was looking inward, all I could find inside myself was just blackness and coldness. "Let's try this," I thought, "and see what happens." I set my book aside. I was alone in my room and I closed my eyes and just thought, "Well, if God is real, how do I picture God?" The thing that came to mind was just whiteness, a silvery whiteness everywhere, all around me, everywhere. So in my mind I reached out, I actually did reach out my hand, and tried to touch it, just to take a little piece of it inside me, and when I touched it in my imagination, and I turned my hand, there was something in my hand. It was like a blue-white star, like a point of light with rays just shining out. I took this little point of God, this infinitesimally tiny part, and I put it to my chest.

As soon as I put it into my chest, something took over my body. It was physical. I felt like something was blowing me up inside. I could feel my skin bulging outward, and I started to gasp for breath. I felt an ecstasy that was—the only way I can describe it is that it was just like a sexual climax, except that there was nothing physical to it and it was better than a sexual climax, infinitely better. It was entirely like a spiritual climax, and I was gasping for breath, and then I was grabbing the bed. This thing had control of me; I mean something took over my body. It was very physical. I was not in control. Something was doing this to me, and I don't know how long it lasted, but probably for about ten seconds. It seemed like a long time.

When it left me, I just wept. I was just stunned. I thought, "What the hell was that?" I mean, it was real. This wasn't just something in my imagination. Something literally grabbed me, something touched me. At first, I was just saying, "Thank you, thank you, thank you, my God, thank you." And the very next thought was "Why me? Why me?" And then the next one was "What do you want from me?" I was just absolutely at a loss for why it was so intense. I was looking for some little thing to help me feel better about the next week. This was incredible, powerful, overwhelming, and I was just holding my chest. I could feel warmth, like a glowing inside me. I could feel warmth and life inside me. It was like there was light inside me where there had been just darkness before. I lay there for about ten minutes, just absolutely stunned, and then I said, "I've got to record this," and I grabbed this notebook and wrote it down, what happened. It was hard to find words for it.

Later that evening the subject of God came up again, and I felt like I had understanding. In physics there's something called the uncertainty principle in quantum mechanics, and there's also something called chaos. Both of them say it's absolutely impossible to control the future; you can only affect the probabilities and never control the future. So all of a sudden it hit me that God is that which determines, of the many possible outcomes, what actually occurs. I thought, "Gee, that's kind of neat. Here is God and physics and quantum mechanics and chaos and the twelve-step program, and it all fits together." In the twelve-step program, see, the first thing you do is to let go of your control and admit that you're powerless over affecting the outcome. Once you abandon that control, you feel this great relief because you've handed it to something else. At the time I didn't understand why my experience was so powerful. I had no idea. I was worrying, "What does God want from me? Why me? Why did God pick *me*? Of all the people to have this powerful an experience, why me?" I could have doubted the earlier little voice in my head as just my imagination, but this was physical. It was palpable. I mean it was unbelievable. It was a complete loss of control over my body, like something entered me. I was totally surprised. I felt panic, like "What's happening? What is this? What's going on?" Yet it also all made sense. Then I started to talk to some other people and began hearing about others who had had powerful experiences. I made it through survivors' week, and it was wonderful, I mean it was a tremendous, tremendous release.

The third week was family week. My counselor turned out to be an extremely incompetent and somewhat vicious person, and family week was absolutely horrible. All they did was confrontation between my wife and my kids and me. There was no healing, there was no positive stuff, it was all negative, and at the end of the week they just left the whole family shattered and torn apart. They left us all just hanging. The strength of my spiritual experience made no sense at the time, but it turns out I needed that strength to get through what was coming in those next two weeks. What was given to me was a knowledge, a personal knowledge, that there is a spiritual side to life. Before it was just a hypothesis, an intellectual exercise, reasoning whether there is a God. The knowledge that I was given was a certainty. It was a personal experience that it's there. It's real, as real as physics is real.

My wife already knew. She always had a deep-seated belief in God. At the end of family week, as I told you, this counselor just had us confronting each other. Mainly them confronting me for an entire week. All this anger, all this frustration was coming out, all this pain, all this remembering of all the things I had done in the past. At the end of that week my wife didn't know what was going to happen, whether we'd still be together or whether the family was going to be destroyed. She saw all this pain in her children. It was completely negative, it was confrontational. So she was lying in bed, and feeling cold and shaking and desperate and fearful for the future, and she felt like something took her hand. It was like a warm hand grabbed her hand. She told me about that later.

These things happen, you know.

A frustrating thing to me was that after I went through all this stuff, I still wasn't cured. I still didn't feel cured when the subject of money came up. I would still feel the lure of using alcohol once in a while. So I found a behavior therapist and went off and on for a year, and he taught me about behavioral psychology. I learned that, OK, it's very nice that I have this understanding, but I'm still also an animal that's been conditioned and until I do some relearning, by taking control instead of avoiding it, I'm going to feel these things. You see, knowing this helps keep everything in perspective. I'm no longer interested in making a lot of money. I have just decided to step down from my position at work, because it's no fun responding to pressure and feeling that I have to be a workaholic to belong to the club. I just want to do my research and have fun. If I make less money, that's fine, I don't care. I just want to have a serene day-to-day life. I don't want to be president some day. What I get excited about now is walking in the woods, just taking in what's there, and celebrating the creation.

Now I feel connections with other people. I find that most people have a shell. With some people I can't see the real person inside them. The shell's just too thick. My colleagues at work, I don't even know where they are in there. All I see is this intellectual shell. The real person hardly ever shows through. But with some people, friends for example, I can see that little kid, that inner self inside them, and when I see that, there's a level of communication there which is just magical. It's like love, just absolutely connected by the soul or souls. I never had that before, except fleetingly with my wife. There was always intellect. My own shell was pretty thick, but not so thick that my wife couldn't see through it. That's what kept us together in spite of the hardships. My wife saw the real me when we were first married, and then she wondered where it went as I became more and more centered on my career. Self-actualization isn't in achieving—it's in peace. It's in contentment and being who you are, celebrating who you are, and knowing who you are. So few people know that.

13

A VOICE IN THE FIREPLACE

In 1960 we had an old freestanding fireplace in the kitchen of an old farmhouse. You could walk around it, and I was walking around it when all of a sudden I heard a voice call my name and say, "All you have to do to be happy is to do what you believe." It was a strange man's voice, nothing that I recognized. Had I believed in God at that point in time, I would have become a born-again Christian. There's just no question about it.

I knew the voice was in my head. My wife and children were there in the family room, but I couldn't say anything to them about it. After all, I'm hearing voices, I'm nuts.

All of a sudden I dropped about ten stories in tension. I felt a quiet, relaxed world, a way of being. I had never realized what a tension-free world was about. My wife lived that way, but I never understood it. I was always a driving, pushing individual. I couldn't have been more surprised. I wondered what had happened.

Now, from that point on, I didn't want to go back to that tense world. I couldn't for anything go back to being the way I was before. The peace and quiet that I had found, there's no way that I could go back, so I started looking at what I believed. I came up with a physical tension signal that told me when I wasn't doing what I believed. The pit of my stomach told me. Then I either followed my belief completely or I changed my belief. A lot of times I didn't want to change my beliefs, and I found some of them I couldn't change. Even if I didn't like the consequences, I still had to follow my belief totally.

Everything revolves around belief, to a major degree. Fact is, I feel that the only difference between animals and humanity is belief. Animals think in a lot of ways, but none of them form thought in a way that it becomes true, or can transfer that trueness to another individual so that it produces similar motivation.

That led me within a very short time into, I call it meditation, but really it's closer to relaxation. I've been meditating or relaxing for forty years now. When I was still working (I've been retired the last twenty-three years), it took me half an hour every morning and night to get down to a low level of tension. Even after doing it at eleven o'clock at night and then sleeping, the well of tension had built up by the next morning. Since I retired, I found that I can drop down to a low level in three to five minutes any time I want to. There just isn't any conflict in my life. That's the whole secret of it. You cannot have a responsible job or raise a family and not have conflict.

What really happened is that the lowered tension level allowed my conscious and unconscious to become totally integrated. That's roughly what happened. Tension prohibits that. They call it man's separation from himself. By doing what I believed, I did away with the tension, and the communications within myself were established for the first time in my life. For the first time in my life I understood my wife and all of the knowledge that she had. She was so wise. Everything that she had always said that I didn't understand now made such wonderful sense to me. She had always known.

I've noticed something about alcohol. You see, my wife always loved me a little bit happy from liquor, because it released a very happy, gregarious person. Alcohol never made me mean or angry as it does so many people. I was only a very happy person. It didn't take much. Just a little bit, and I was happier. Even if I got a little bit tight, I was just happy about everything; everybody was my friend. Now, after this experience, I quit drinking for ten years, because I fully believed that alcohol made it more difficult for me to lead the life that I wanted to lead, to follow my beliefs totally. If you release the inhibitions of some of your beliefs, then you're not following them in a sense. Anyhow, she missed that, she really did. I came back gradually. I still don't like alcohol, but I love wine and some beer.

So, as I say, I've had a lot of success with my photography, landscapes. Sometimes, like at a reception for four hours or so, I drink more wine than I intended to, and I notice that when I drink now I never get happy anymore. I don't know what it means, but that's something. I have somehow killed the happy-go-lucky person inside me that used to be released by alcohol. That's the best way I can explain it. Now I just get sleepy. Once after I drank too much wine, I didn't remember coming home. Now I drink one glass of wine, period. It isn't worth the risk to me and to someone else.

Total honesty is one of the biggest changes that happened. Before I had that experience, I wasn't too dishonest but I would sneak. The supply room had all kinds of goodies, and I just took them, and let other people do it too. After that experience, I couldn't do it. I had to stop it. Before that, if I went into a store and gave somebody a five dollar bill and I got ten dollars back in change, I thought, "Well, I won this time. They probably won from me last time." I can't do that anymore. I surprise more cashiers by saying "You better count that again." I can't do it. I cause conflict in me if I do it, that's the whole reason. It's a selfish reason for being honest. As long as I'm honest, I don't develop any conflict or any tension within myself.

I used to run everywhere I went. Afterward I slowed down and I walk very slowly and relaxed. One of the biggest things is that, after I changed, I listened to people. When you listen to people, they enjoy it and they feel much better for being listened to. You're not adding to a conversation at all. You just sit and listen to them. I quit telling people what to do. I still suggest something to somebody once, but I never say it twice. I never get on people's backs, and they appreciate this to no end.

My small son would always come to his mother at bedtime and take her by the hand. He wanted her to take him up to bed, never me. Within three months after I had changed, he came to me and wanted me to take him to bed. It was the most emotional, thrilling experience in my life.

Another important change—and this did not occur at once; it happened, I would say, over three to four years—is that I changed from a conscious, thinking, acting person to a totally unconscious reacting individual. People would come into my office with a problem. They'd tell me what the problem was, and my reaction was always the same. I would settle back in my chair, tilt it back and close my eyes and feel, and an answer would present itself ninety-nine percent of the time, which was right at least ninety percent of the time. I never thought up answers. I switched from conscious hypothesis making to unconscious feeling. I went from a conceptualizer to a feeler.

Socializing changed, too. I went from a very dependent person to a very independent person. Unfortunately, unless it is a true emotional friend, I am no longer content with mob or group participation. I still do some of it, but the people in it don't really interest me. I'm separated from the group as far as interest is concerned, yet I try not to let them know that. One of the biggest problems that I have today is I accept help reluctantly. That's not good. I didn't realize that at times you need to do it for the other person. I do that with my family, accept help, but it's difficult for me. I'm very independent.

This change has lasted, no question about it. Forty years. I have seen sensitivity groups come together and find a peaceful orientation, but most of the people drift away. They have a slight experience of peace, but by the time they get back to work and the rest of life, it's all gone. Not so with my experience If anything, each day you might say it's stronger.

14

AT PECOS

About six years ago I went on a retreat at the Pecos Benedictine monastery, and I didn't have any particular ideas about what to expect. I wasn't looking for anything in particular; just wanted to have some quiet time, something like that. Anyway, at that retreat, I had an emotional born-again experience—experiencing Christ on the cross and knowing that he died for my sins. It was just sort of like a vision, something in my head, that I had been there as He was on the cross, and walked there among the crowd in the dirt and the dust and the hot sun and all the rest of it, and I experienced what was happening. I wouldn't call it a vision or a light. It was like I was there the afternoon of Christ's crucifixion, as a part of the crowd, watching everything that was going on. I could get inside all of them: the people who were there mocking Him, the Roman soldiers, the people who were His family, His apostles. It was like I was experiencing all their different feelings, how they were relating to what was happening to Him on the cross. What I regret now is that I didn't write that down, because a lot of it has sort of faded.

I felt a great sense of remorse and repentance, and at the same time a feeling of forgiveness for my sins. It was internal; it was in my head. There were a lot of tears and a lot of regret for the things I had done, but it was like a great weight had been lifted. I didn't feel as though I had to feel any more remorse for what I had done. It was just important to start from that day and do things differently.

The experience itself wasn't particularly remarkable, other than the emotional experience of feeling a great sense of sadness and a great sense of relief at the same time. It was a kind of cleansing. The repentance that I felt in my heart was a gift from God. In other words, God allowed me to be truly repentant. Immediately I felt as though I could dispense with those things that were troubling in my personal life: my inclination to spend too much money, or drink too much alcohol, or stay up too late, or get involved in things that were wasting my time. I felt as though those burdens had been removed and I didn't have a need to do them anymore. Eventually, I had a feeling of lightness and exhaustion—and tears.

It was the Holy Spirit working through me, and it was my acceptance of my Catholic faith. At some point, I don't know exactly when I made the choice, but I must have said something like "What do you want me to do, Lord? I'm yours. Where do I go from here?" Afterward I spoke to a priest from Puerto Rico who happened to be there just for a short time, and he told me of a similar thing that had happened to him about three years previously, in his relationship with the Lord and his own struggle with remaining in the priesthood.

As a result of the experience afterward I felt differently. I went to AA for thirty days. I knew that I drank too much. I went to a least one meeting a day for a month, and I never drank again after that, which was about six years ago. I persisted and went for thirty days, but by the time the month was over I didn't feel a need for it. I felt more of a bond and connection with people in my church than I did in going to AA. If people want to pursue AA, I think that's fine, that it's a valid thing to do.

My experience changed my perspective on my church life and my family and my wife. I just felt differently about things. One thing that struck me about the whole retreat, when they talked about midlife crisis, they said that the only way you can avoid midlife crisis is to develop a mature spirituality as you get into midlife. Basically, until I was forty years old, religion for me was like a social responsibility. You know, you went to church, you did certain things with your kids, you educated them in Catholic school, or whatever. Now I had a different feeling about that. I just continued to become more involved in church activities. For example, we regularly go into the Bernalillo county jail for Bible study and to do services. This is something that never would have occurred to me in the more hedonistic type of lifestyle I had had previously. I didn't realize that people living in a situation like prison have so much to give me. I often get more out of it than I think they do.

Earlier, I had been divorced and remarried. When my oldest daughter was about seventeen and a senior in high school, they found a lump in her thyroid and suspected it might be cancer. I flew to where the girls lived with my first wife, to be there for her surgery. That was about two years after the experience at Pecos. I remember my ex-wife saying to me, "There is something different about you." I didn't tell her anything about—you know—the experience, or being a born-again Christian or anything like that. That's all she said: "There's something different about you." She didn't elaborate, and I didn't ask her anything more about it.

The retreat made me realize that belief in God is always a mystery that will never be understood, and part of it is faith. You just have to make that decision. For about forty years of my life, it was like I had sat on the wall or the fence, never making a commitment one way or the other and expecting to live in two worlds, as the Bible says—pursuing the worldly things and trying to pursue the spiritual things at the same time. They don't mix, and you just sort of waste your time, spin your wheels. That's my feeling about it and the way I look at it now.

My wife and I had always done things that we found interesting. We were looking for the great answer—you know, what life is all about. We had gone to a number of different things, searching. You know, it's funny that you use the word "quantum" change in your project here, because one of the things I remember that we did was to go hear a speaker who was a physicist in Ann Arbor. He was talking about quantum mechanics and physics and its relationship with spirituality and God. Both of us had an interest in that kind of thing for many years, that sort of philosophical intellectual approach to spirituality.

I had never experienced anything like this before, even through the use of drugs, where you have a false sense of enlightenment. It to me seemed valid and beyond all expectations that I ever had for something like that. Yet it was extremely simple. I guess a lot of it had to do with giving up my own defenses, my intellectualizing about it, and letting my emotional side come through. I'm not an emotional person, and I tend to be analytical.

Before this, hedonistic or selfish pursuits were important to me.

I hung out with a different type of people. Before this, I worked in research where I hardly ever dealt with people. I dealt mostly with animals, and I was real happy with that. Now I'm working in a clinic where I have an opportunity to talk to people who are really messed up on drugs, and I look for some way to encourage them to get some semblance of regularity or spirituality in their life. Even though it's discouraging at times, I do it anyway. I'm not a counselor, but I see the clients regularly when they come in.

Religion is the center of my life now. It's not compartmentalized, like just going to church on Sunday. My church life is all through everything that I do. I consider what Scripture says or try to consider what Scripture says about all decisions in my life: in the way I raise my children, in the way I relate to my wife, the way I relate to my employer. Before, I wouldn't have any second thoughts about trying to get paid for more hours than I worked—that kind of thing.

There's a lot more to becoming sober than to just stop drinking. It's only part of it, to not be affected by drugs or alcohol. The rest of it is being able to free yourself from all those other bondages that hold you back from being open, sincere in relationships, especially with your wife. You have to work at those things. In the past I behaved in a selfish manner, not even realizing I was being selfish, and not realizing that I had anything to be repentant for. It was the furthest thing from my mind.

Now that I feel that my future is assured, I feel comfortable even with the mistakes I make now. I regret making mistakes, but I don't get immobilized. I don't feel as though I have to use drugs, or turn to drink, or something like that. I feel that prayer can give me an answer, and if it's not immediate, I also understand that eventually it'll become clear.

Before this, my Catholic faith was a veil of tears. You can seek absolution for your sins, but you don't expect a life change; you just expect to be forgiven for your sins and go on about your way in your own compulsive destructive behavior. That's how I was.

I would say that this experience was the hand of God and it was timed at the right point, where I could have ended up like some of the folks I see in the jail now. I also realize how far we are from despair. No matter how bad our situation is—where I live, whatever I have to put up with—it's nothing. Nothing would be as terrible as separation from God.

15

TRAMPOLINE

This happened fourteen years ago, when I was in my twenties. I was teaching a gymnastics trampoline class. We were four minutes into class, and I was demonstrating a trick for the students, a double back flip. In the demonstration, one of the students asked to see it again. I'd already demonstrated it twice, and the third time was the charm. I'd put my feet on the trampoline and I'd open up and I'd see the trampoline. I'd explained to him that when you open up you'll see the trampoline below you, and to spot where you put your feet. When I opened up this time, I was looking at the roof, so I knew there was something out of whack. I landed on my head instead of my feet, and I knew as soon as I hit the trampoline that I'd done something to my neck, because I couldn't move and I was totally numb.

When I hit the trampoline, I can't say that I heard a voice actually saying "Be still," but I just somehow heard that: "Be still." And then a warmth came over my body. It was like coming in out of the cold and somebody who's nice and warm just grabbing you and holding you in their arms. It was just a warmth, like being in good strong warm hands. That's when I realized, as soon as that feeling and that voice or whatever it was came to me, that God in some way was saying "I'm in control. OK, now you take control of the physical circumstances. I'm in control of everything else, but you take control of the physical circumstances. Look around. Check out what's going on. See how you feel physically. Tell everybody else what needs to be done. I'll take care of the rest."

I'd had emergency medical technician training, so I knew from the total numbness that they shouldn't move me. Plus in gymnastics, I'd seen accidents. You don't touch somebody until you get a person with higher medical expertise to check them out. So I told the students not to get on the trampoline, not to touch me. Go get the athletic trainer and call the paramedics. They were there in minutes.

I kind of had fun with the paramedics. One of the assistant trainers told them it was a major neck injury. I heard one of the paramedics say, "I wonder if we've got a live one or not." So I closed my eyes, and I could feel one of the paramedics crawling up on the trampoline. He slowly made his way toward me, and when he was fairly close I opened my eyes and told him, "I think I broke my neck." He was kind of stunned, and he said, "We've got a live one here who knows what's happening!"

After a couple of seconds of silence, he said, "What do you think we should be doing?" I said, "I need to get on a backboard, need to be stabilized." He said, "OK. Do you want us to turn you over?" I was lying semi-facedown on the trampoline. I told him, "No, I'd rather be placed on the backboard in the position that I'm in and stabilized and bagged off in this position until I get to the hospital." Just in case there was major breakage or damage, I wasn't risking any other sort of movement of the spinal cord.

So then they put me on the backboard in the position that I was in, took me off, and by that time the ambulance was there. In the ambulance the paramedics were playing mental games with me, to make sure I was really conscious and alert to what I was talking about. They asked me what hospital I wanted to go to. I told them the one I wanted, since I knew that they had a good spinal cord, neurological program there. Then the person sitting right beside me started giving the wrong directions—the directions to a different hospital—and I said, "No, that's not the right hospital!" He said, "OK, St. Joseph's, that means we have to go out to Gibson and San Mateo." I said, "No, that's Lovelace. Go down Central to University and take University over to Grand and down Grand." "Oh, you want to go to Presbyterian!" "No!—to St. Joseph's." Then he gave directions to still a different hospital, and I corrected him. It was an ongoing verbal sparring to make sure that I was staying alert and conscious.

So I kind of took charge, but once I was in the hospital I had to rely on what the doctors were saying. Still, I chose how I was going to respond to what was happening. I had to ask them, because they were talking in technical terms, "Can you bring that down to lay-men's language so I can understand what is happening?" I wanted to know what the consequences might be. I wanted to know what was going on, so that I could understand and go on with it and see what the next step was. I was trying to understand what they were doing, why they were doing what they were doing, poking me and moving me and standing me on my head, and all the other tests they were running on me. Gymnastics is an individual sport where you're mainly competing against yourself. You become a perfectionist and want to know "What am I doing, why am I doing this, and if I'm not doing it right, why am I not doing it right?"—total understanding in a language that's understandable. It's soul searching, answering everything, just wanting to have total control over virtually all that is going on, or to be able to understand why you do not have total control.

After about seven hours, the doctor came in and told me the worst case—that I would be paralyzed from the neck down. I hadn't actually damaged my spinal cord, but I had dislocated three vertebrae that had severely bruised it. The swelling would go down in twenty-four to forty-eight hours, and then they would know how much damage had been done from lack of blood supply. He said he couldn't promise anything and I should be prepared for the worst.

In a split second, I went from being a very, very active person—one who needed twenty-eight hours a day to get everything done and running full blast driving here and there and going everywhere all the time—to just not being able to move. So I began thinking "What are my options now?" I was thankful to still be alive and OK. So what options am I going to have now in going on with my life? I guess I'll take it one step at a time and find out what is going to be available to me.

It was about a week afterward that I first really put it into words when I was talking with one of the nurses, that it was like I was starting my life all over again, being born all over again, except this time my mind was fully developed and I'd be learning to live all over again.

Everything that I knew before, I was going to have to throw out the window. Essentially it was OK, starting all over, starting from scratch and finding out what I can and cannot do, learning how to do the things that I need to do to function as an individual.

For the first several weeks it was kind of a flood of information. My mind was running through "OK, how do I adapt to this situation? How do I adapt to that?"—almost deprogramming my mind from everything that I had been doing to letting it be open, opening it up to be able to be taught.

It wasn't like a religious conversion, really. I'm a Christian and I have been through that, but it was totally different from that. It was a total physical conversion from a very active person to somebody with no activity whatsoever for a week or two. Then I slowly began to get movement back in my arms, and the best way I can put it is that it was like being born with a fully developed mind. I know I want to feed myself, so how do I do it? How am I going to make my livelihood? Never having dealt with anybody with a disability who was out in the workforce, that was one of the little questions that came up at first. Before this happened, I had said one of those things you really shouldn't ever say: "I'll never, never work behind a desk in my life."

Everything, virtually everything, that I had been doing in my life, I was going to have to put on the back bookshelf of my mind and be a resource to draw from for problem solving later on in life. Just start anew and take it one step at a time. The first ones are going to be small, baby steps, and then maybe some larger ones, and then maybe a breakthrough or bigger steps, or maybe a step backward.

My spiritual grounding was very, very helpful. I knew that there was a bigger picture, that God had things in control. This hadn't happened for no reason. God would use it in some way that I had no idea of at that time. I knew that there was a plan for this in some way, and it would turn out to be for the best. I saw quite a few other people in the hospital at that time who felt like things had happened to them for no reason at all, who felt just adrift in the universe and stuck out in the middle of nowhere for no reason. They wondered why they should even continue on. My faith helped me to get through this and keep moving on with my life.

That experience relieved me of a huge mental burden. I had rushed around at such a fast pace, I was trying to be perfect, and because of that I took on a lot more responsibility than I needed to and didn't delegate any responsibilities. At times it tended to be very burdensome. I would let other people do the job, but then I would go back and go over it again to make sure it was done correctly. It wasn't that I didn't trust them. I just wanted to make sure everything was done exactly right. No stone was left unturned. Now, up to the point of the accident, I didn't see myself doing that. I didn't realize that I was doing that. Other people may have and they didn't say anything, but I myself didn't dwell on it. That's probably why I was running on a twenty-eight-hour or thirty-hour day, trying to get everything done in twenty-four. It was a burden. I never felt like I could get it all done on time. Then, after the accident, I realized that I don't have to worry about this other stuff. When I was in the hospital, I realized, "Oh, this is to stop, slow down and smell the roses." I don't have to do it all myself. I can stop, smell the roses, and let other people do what they need to do.

I wasn't really hard on other people, but I was harder on myself than anybody else. It was the perfectionist within myself. I was lenient with other people; they could make mistakes and I would fix it. I still find myself falling into it at times, the workaholic type of attitude. When I do I just take a couple days off, back off, take a few deep breaths, and say, "OK, you're taking everything too seriously. Let the people do what they're supposed to do." I can see it much more vividly now. Sometimes I come home after work totally exhausted, physically and mentally. I know when I'm at that point I've taken on too much. I try to get it across to everybody—no matter whether they've had a similar experience or anything, just a normal everyday person—that's the way life is. It's not a matter of know-it-all and everything, but meet each day by itself because there's going to be something new each day that we can learn from, that we grab hold of and learn about, and a problem that comes up that we have to learn to deal with. Accept the challenges that the day presents.

The slowing down of my lifestyle allowed me to see a lot more of the beauty in the world, just to take time to see and to analyze it. To see people and not judge them on a quick first impression, not judge them for what they do right then, but to see them more compassionately in a longer-term picture. It makes for a whole lot nicer world.

One of my little hobbies is writing poems. After the accident, I lived with my parents, and my bedroom looked out onto a golf course. One of the first poems I wrote after the accident was of watching the golfers as they played, walking on the golf course, walking up the fairway and taking a wood out and hitting it and getting mad and stomping off and running off. If they'd just stop to see and just take it easy, take a deep breath, just relax and enjoy the *game* of golf! Sure they're out there doing a sport, trying to be competitive and doing the best they can, but it also can be so relaxing, if they'd take the time, just seeing all the green and the beautiful forest all around them. I know I did the same thing, and I probably missed out on a lot of beauty. I missed out on just seeing a lot of things that I probably could have seen, had I taken the time and slowed down in the things that I was doing.

What's changed in me? I'm the same as far as my way of thinking about things, analyzing things, but I do it at a slower pace now. I'm not so quick to make a decision or make a judgment until I've done more analyzing of the situation. I guess the other part of it is that I don't feel that I have a negative attitude. I really try to be positive, see the positive side of anything that's going on. My spirituality is deeper and more enhanced. I understand better our dependence on God, and God's control over things that we don't understand.

I also found out who my real friends were. The people who said then that they were my friends, for the first month or so they came down visiting me all the time at the hospital. It slowly died out, slowly but surely there were fewer and fewer, down to two or three close friends who really stuck with me all the way through it. They have moved away, but we still stay in touch on a regular basis. I found out what the real meaning of "friend" is.

PART IV

REFLECTIONS

16

AFTER

Lead on, Spirit! Lead on! The night is waning fast, and
it is precious time to me, I know.
—EBENEZER SCROOGE, to the Ghost of Christmas Yet to Come
in Charles Dickens, *A Christmas Carol*

One thing that distinguishes a quantum change from
other insights and mystical experiences is the profound and lasting
effect that it has on the person. It is not just a change in a discrete
behavior, like stopping smoking or becoming more talkative. When
we asked, "What was different after your experience?" a representa-
tive response was "Everything." The transformations described were
usually at the level of personality, of core guiding principles, of the
person's way of perceiving and understanding self and reality:

*I still have trials and tribulations, and the gas bill isn't going down.
Reality is the same. Life is the same. It's how I look at things and
how things are pointed out to me that has changed. Life has not
changed at all. People are still people. They still drive crazy in
rush hour, and I still get angry with them, although I'm a little
more patient with them now. Things have not changed per se, but
I'm totally different than I was. I am not the person I used to be, in
any shape or form.*

Change sweeps through the person's behavior, emotions, attitudes, values, and thought processes. To be sure, for some people the changes were much broader than for others, but virtually all would say that what changed was "me." There was something about the person's sense of self that was fundamentally different afterward.

We weren't sure exactly what to expect when we designed our questions about life after quantum change. We weren't even sure what to ask. Obviously we wanted to know how the experience had affected their lives and relationships, and we were fascinated with the opportunity to gain a longer-term perspective than is found in the initial change stories. What was Scrooge like ten years later? We found that in interesting ways, our storytellers seemed to have become more similar to one another after quantum change. They started out quite diverse—so much so that we found it difficult to paint a portrait of the "typical" candidate for quantum change. Afterward, though, they began to look more alike.

EMOTIONS

Nearly every quantum change story described substantial changes in emotionality, and not merely during the experience itself. The transformation left the person different emotionally in a way that endured across the years. Often this involved release from longstanding patterns of negative emotion. A woman who had been severely abused by her father explained her emotional change in this way:

> How has all this changed me? Well, whatever happens, I'm just at peace. I'm not afraid anymore, and I don't think of myself as ugly and dirty and trashy. I'm not afraid of my father. I'm secure and self-assured. I have the patience of a saint now! Before I wanted everything right now, and of course that doesn't happen. My outlook on men has changed. I've learned that everyone has good in them. Before, I had no feeling of good in anyone. In fact, people were the ugliest things ever created. I think I'm more lenient because of these experiences. I'm more understanding. I hate to say this, but I can understand my father. I can have sympathy and understanding for him. I don't hate him. I think he's very sick, warped, terribly misguided. It depends on how you look at things, how you think of this life, how you perceive why you are here. I'm not filled with the an-

ger I had, and I can have a lot more compassion, even for those who treated me badly. I'm not saying I like them. I'm not saying I'll ever forgive. I will never forgive my father for what he did to me, the ugliness and the horror, but I will say I do understand now that he's a sick person. Before I just felt he was evil, that he should be put to death, tortured, mutilated. Now that's gone. I'm at peace.

Another woman spoke of the lifting of life-threatening depression:

I used to be real suicidal before. I thought, "Who cares if you die? You just come back as somebody else." I believed in reincarnation and that it would be cool to go through death and experience it and then come back and remember. Now I'm very comfortable knowing that whatever happens in the future I will be with God eternally, and it's real peaceful to think about that. I don't want to rush it, but I have no fear of death. I guess security is the word.

Release from disabling fear was another common theme:

Before this experience, I was very much afraid. I was afraid not to believe in God. I was afraid of being punished. I followed all the rules because I was scared of what would happen if I didn't. I was afraid of everything, even afraid of God. When my son was sick, I felt like I was being punished. I really felt like I had done something wrong in my life and God was punishing me. This experience changed me in the sense that there's really nothing in this world that I'm afraid of now. I don't mean that in a happy-go-lucky way, like I would go get drunk and drive home because I'm not afraid of dying. I just mean that I'm not afraid. I'm not intimidated by authoritative people. People with authority don't scare me anymore. I started up this little company, and I'm going to be very successful in it. I look for a future of being in a position where my little company will be solid and put the groceries on the table, and then I can do something a lot more humanitarian. What that is I don't know yet, but that's my goal. It's like I've got to make this company work so my family will be OK, and then I can do something that's important to my heart. I'm a very determined and courageous person now, very responsible. I don't feel intimidated by anything. I'm not even afraid of my own death. I'm not. It's not like I look forward to it, but I'm just not afraid. It's like there's really nothing that frightens

*me. I know some bad things will come. That's all right. I'll deal
with them when they get here. I try to help everyone I can. I'm
more positive now. I'm confident now that I can deal with whatever
comes my way. I try to inspire others, when I hear that they are
down. I try to instill that in my children most of all. I feel really
lucky that I get to live my life like this. I'm no longer afraid, and
that's a beautiful way to live. It really is.*

It was not merely a matter of such negative feelings being removed. Rather, it was clear from people's accounts that they had
been replaced by an enduring sense of calm, peacefulness, hope, security, and inner strength. That theme is evident in all of the epiphany stories in Part III. This emotional calming seems to be particularly characteristic of the mystical, epiphany type of quantum
change.

PRIORITIES

Although quantum changers often answer, "Everything," when
asked what changed, in fact many aspects of the person do stay
the same. What seems to shift, though, is how the person understands and perceives reality. The person's core values change and
become clearer.

*I am just seeing the brightness in the world, the order of things and
how it's supposed to be, as opposed to seeing the discord and dis-
harmony. It's seeing that everything is as it should be right now. I
think I had what is described in the Big Book [of AA] as a complete
psychic change. My motivations and my whole sense of direction in
life have changed. My values changed. What I thought was important changed. I just completely shifted gears. It's given me a sense
of purpose and direction I never had before, a real meaningful purpose in life. I'd always sought that before, and I'd been searching
different avenues but never found exactly what I was supposed to
be doing. I've tried a lot of different things, a lot of different jobs,
traveled a lot, had lots of experiences in my life. Yet always there
was that kind of restless searching, searching. Now I feel like I
know exactly what I'm supposed to do.*

It is not that values were slightly modified or amended. Rather, the person's value system was often turned upside down. Think of Scrooge. Things that had seemed important before the experience abruptly dropped in significance, and what had previously seemed worthless suddenly became precious. Using a structured card-sorting method, we asked people to describe their values before and after their quantum change. Listed in the table below is how women and men described their top twelve (of fifty) values before their experience and now. (A longer list of values in our current card sort is provided in the Appendix to this book.)

There were common "big winners" and "big losers" among the fifty values we queried. Values that had been last became first, and what had once headed the list fell to the bottom. The biggest single gain was in the priority given to spirituality, which rose from the bottom third to first place for men and third place for women. Both men and women also reflected large increases in the value they placed on forgiveness, generosity, God's will, growth, honesty, humility, loving, and personal peace, all of which were reported in the bottom half of priorities before quantum change. The valuing of monetary wealth fell from first to last place for men and dropped thirty ranks for women. For both genders, values previously given higher priority fell toward the bottom of the list: physical attractiveness, authority, career, fitting in, independence, popularity, and romance (also see the Appendix).

Twelve Most Highly Valued Personal Characteristics
(ranked from among 50)

	Men		Women	
	Before	After	Before	After
1.	Wealth	Spirituality	Family	Growth
2.	Adventure	Personal peace	Independence	Self-esteem
3.	Achievement	Family	Career	Spirituality
4.	Pleasure	God's will	Fitting in	Happiness
5.	Be respected	Honesty	Attractiveness	Generosity
6.	Family	Growth	Knowledge	Personal peace
7.	Fun	Humility	Self-control	Honesty
8.	Self-esteem	Faithfulness	Be loved	Forgiveness
9.	Freedom	Forgiveness	Happiness	Health
10.	Attractiveness	Self-esteem	Wealth	Creativity
11.	Popularity	Loving	Faithfulness	Loving
12.	Power	Intimacy	Safety	Family

In other ways, women and men became more similar in their values, moving from opposite extremes toward each other. Men became less macho and materialistic, with major drops in the valuing of achievement, adventure, comfort, fame, fun, power, and being respected—all things that were less initially valued by women. Women's priorities moved closer to men's by a relatively greater drop in emphasis on traditional feminine values: fitting in, faithfulness to others, safety, and self-control. Similarly, men more closely matched women's values after quantum change by relative increases in priority given to caring for others, faithfulness to others, monogamy, helpfulness, intimacy, safety, and self-control. Though family remained high on both lists, the centrality of family increased for men while it decreased for women. In sum, both moved away from the stereotypic gender roles represented in popular media and advertising and toward common and compassionate values and a cherishing of the present. Here is an example:

> I ponder at times what I used to see in the kick from alcohol. I get a lot of that now from natural things. I have found that a sunset, a walk in the moonlight, aromas along the path in the bosque give me more pleasure than I ever got from a buzz. Maybe it's a heightened awareness of the short time we have, all of us.

BEHAVIOR

Rather than being limited to circumscribed behaviors, quantum change typically involves positive shifts or even turnabouts in a broad range of attitudes and behaviors. A common one is the sudden lifting of ingrained habitual behavior that had been exerting destructive effects for many years:

> We used to drink and carouse and do awful things, sexual perversions and a lot of pornographic stuff that we'd been involved with all our life. It's amazing that we weren't caught. I lost all desire to do that ten years ago. Before that encounter, well, I was just so different. Now it's so funny when I talk with women at church in small groups and they may talk about their drug days, I'll say, "Oh, yeah, we used it," and they'll say, "You used to do that? You don't look like the type!" Both my husband and I have this torrid past, but

now we look to other people as if we fit into the mold of the typical Christian and have always been very straight.

Another woman wrote to us:

I had tried desperately and sincerely to stop drinking, but in my heart I knew there was a chance that I couldn't do it. It seemed beyond my control. That morning, however, I awoke from a terrible nightmare, and as I became awake enough to understand where I was, I knew with absolute certainty that I would never drink again. It has been almost a year and a half now, and I still feel exactly the same way. As a bonus, my mind feels at ease and life is wonderful to me for the first time in over forty-five years. I've tried to explain this experience to a few people, but of course, unless a person has been through it, it's impossible to understand.

Many quantum changers had not been vexed by addiction, however, and release from habit and desire is only part of the picture. The changes were more widespread. Participants told us that they started taking care of themselves in many ways. They lost weight, established a more stable lifestyle, drove more patiently, and took time for simple pleasures. Some became actively involved in religion. Others practiced a newfound spirituality outside organized religion through private prayer and meditation. Some for the first time devoted regular time to community service. There were changes, too, in how they spent their time. Pastimes that had filled much of their time before—watching TV, shopping, playing computer games, housecleaning—were replaced by new priorities having to do with spirituality, forgiveness, and personal growth and peace.

RELATIONSHIPS

Many changes were also apparent in relationships. From a subjective standpoint, there was an increased sense of compassion and trust toward others, linked in part to the perception that all humans are deeply interrelated and part of the same whole. In relationships themselves, several themes were common. One was a desire for deeper friendships and an impatience with superficial conversation and relationships:

I have very deep relationships with people now, long lasting and deep. When friends have something that is troubling them, they usually seek me out. I don't have a lot of just casual relationships. Even if we don't spend a lot of time together, the time we spend is profound. What people say about me is that they can think with me, that they feel smart when they're with me, and can talk about things they see. They feel like they can see things that they don't normally see and can talk about them.

Disturbed family relationships were common in the background of those who told us their stories, and here, too, there were changes. Some marriages ended, while others were renewed and enriched. Longstanding issues with family were often resolved for the quantum changer, though not always for others in the family. Often there came an emotional detachment from family dynamics that paradoxically provided space for more positive attachments to grow within the family:

In terms of my family, things have changed. I love my family and I'm detached from them, I'm not hooked in with them. I'm not cut off from them or anything like that, but they say when I'm around it's different, and people can be themselves or can feel: "We can say what's on our mind when you're around." When they thought I wasn't going to come for Christmas, they said, "No, you have to be there!" So I've actually become a kind of leader emotionally, in the areas of love and connection and fun and joy. I guess it's a deeper connection.

Partner and parent relationships were also transformed over time:

This had quite an effect on how I am with my family. My mother is dead now, but when the changes started, I was able to make peace with her before she died. We became friends. I had always hated her. I don't like to use that word, because I don't hate anybody now, but I hated her then because she wouldn't help me. She didn't believe me about the abuse. Years later, I found out that she did believe me, but because of her position in the community, she wouldn't give that up for her daughter. She was the woman of the hour, the woman of the year, lunch with the governor. All that meant a lot more to her than her own daughter, but I was able to make peace with my mother. I always wanted to be the best mother that I never had, and I turned out to be. I have a wonderful daughter who thinks I'm great.

Another woman told us:

I don't really have an explanation for it. I just know it happened. It gave me a courage to deal with some of the marital problems. I went back to school and got a master's. There were things I had been afraid to do, to really be what I wanted to be, and I wasn't afraid of that anymore. I was not afraid to take on certain responsibilities. There was a confidence there that I just didn't have before. I didn't recognize that so much immediately as I did maybe three or six months later, when I had made some decisions to put some of these things in motion.

And my daughter made a turnaround. It seemed that when I let up on her, or because of the experience (or both), she and I got along better. Several months later, for my birthday—I loved a particular blueberry cake donut that a little local bakery made, and she bought me two dozen. She told me to freeze them for my birthday. It was the first kind thing that she had done for me in quite a while. This thing just popped into my mind, but there was a big change for her, too. Now, I'm not saying that her behavior changed completely overnight, because it didn't. It took another year before she seemed to get her act really together. She now works with children and is a beautiful person, but back then I didn't think she was so beautiful. [She laughs.] We have a special relationship now, she and I. It's almost like ESP.

I never really talked to her about my experience. It's just that at some point I moved out of that dogmatic parent role toward a supportive friend type of relationship. I'll always be the mother, you know, but it became very different and we did things together. She went on to college, and we used to discuss some of the things we had read with each other.

My son in college developed alcoholism and I, for myself and for him, began going to Al-Anon. So when he had to be hospitalized after a suicide attempt, I was able to in a sense love him and support him yet be somewhat detached. I was able and willing to say to him, "You have to leave." Sometimes it's almost as if it's not me who is saying and doing what I know to be the appro-

*priate thing, not only for myself but for them. He didn't like be-
ing kicked out of the house, but he could say to me after two
years of sobriety, "That was one of the best things you ever did
for me, Mom." That still gives me chill bumps.*

    *I think I've always been a different person since that experi-
ence always; I had people, particularly after I started back in
school, say to me, "You have changed! You're different!" My husband was a very strong, powerful person, and I think that I had
been sort of living my life as his extension for years. All of a
sudden I wasn't his extension anymore. I was me. I had a sort of
a selfhood or just confidence, and that was wonderful. It was a
freedom. It's like I know what I want to do. I don't compromise
myself. I have a kind of homing device if I get off a little bit. I'm
not saying that there haven't been bad times, or doubt and fear,
but that homing device has always been there.*

Quantum change never seemed to sour a previously solid relationship, at least not from the storyteller's perspective. Some prior
friendships fell away, sometimes because after quantum change they
were perceived to be shallow, other times because prior friends had
difficulty with the relationship intensity that followed the experience.

SPIRITUALITY

Spirituality, as we've seen, soared from the bottom to the top of the
priority list among those men who had experienced a quantum
change and to third place for women quantum changers. In the stereotypic religious conversion, a person moves from no real faith to
zealous involvement in a religion. Although we heard a few such stories, more often the change was to a secure individual spirituality
that might or might not include involvement in organized religion:

    *I've become very spiritual, although I'm not a follower of any reli-
gion. I seek out mentors. I feel like I've been being trained for something somehow, like there's been this series of lessons. My latest lesson in just the last year is a fine-tuning of this difference between
"my will" and "Thy will." Now, I'm not a religious person, but
there's something about "Thy will." It's that there's something hap-*

*pening I don't know about but I can tap into, I can surrender to it. I
get in trouble when I try to impose my will, what I think should
happen, on that process. I have no idea what the future holds. I
don't actually care. I have no fear of death at all. I feel really safe.*

Others, like this nurse, found that the experience transformed their
spirituality within their religious traditions:

*Eventually, as a Christian, I came to accept who I was, that God
loves me. The difference between religion and spirituality, in my
mind, is that in any church you go to what you hear is: "God loves
you if . . . . . . God loves you if you give ten percent; God loves you
if you are straight, not gay; God loves you if you don't believe in
abortion; God loves you if." To me, after that experience, spirituality is: God loves me, period, unconditionally and no ifs. It's there. I
can tap into it. It's for me.*

Many had been no stranger to religion. Some had had a strong
religious upbringing, with either positive or negative experiences,
but found in their quantum change a new depth of spirituality:

*I feel I have become a more spiritual person. My mother was Cath-
olic. I came from a large Catholic family, so when I was with her
side of the family we went to Mass, we prayed the rosary, and I always thought that was kind of fun. My father was a stern Presbyterian. When we'd get ready to go to church on Sunday morning, if
Mother happened to drive we went to the Catholic church. I chose
when I was about fifteen to become a Presbyterian. I went to a Bap-
tist college and married a Methodist. I had a spiritual mentor who
was an Episcopal priest. So I've had a mulligan stew of all this religious input.*

*I don't recall ever having a religious experience like hearing
God call me or having a particular insight during a time of
prayer or devotion. I've never had a problem with believing that
God exists. I tried to approach it at certain times from an intellectual perspective, looking at the religions of the world and
reading Greek mythology. I always come around to this same
thing, basically still the tenets that we see in Judaism and Christianity.*

In this experience I've gotten a confirmation for what I feel is truth. I pray every day. I have a quiet time when I first get up in the morning, and I read Scriptures. I have a series of lectures and articles that I reread from my Episcopal priest friend, and I use other devotional materials. I pray for myself and for other people. It's meaningful to me. Sometimes I pray the rosary just to feel the connection with my Catholic ancestors. They were good to me. They loved me.

Maybe what happened to me was God. I don't know, but it didn't really bother me as to what it was. It just was. I've never had that kind of thing happen again. I do talk to God: "I don't understand this, God," or "You'll have to speak louder," or "Your will be done, not mine; You know better than I." I feel we have a good relationship. God slaps my hand every now and then, but that's OK. I just shriek and say, "That's not fair!"

I am very grateful for it, wherever it came from: something somewhere, God perhaps, whatever out there cared enough. When you get that kind of assurance and you begin to see how it is reflected in new attitudes and new behavior, then you see that it's going to be OK. There's no doubt. I can't tell you all the fallout from that night, but it was good.

Others were raised without a religious tradition and found spirituality anew.

I have absolute faith that there's a God. No doubt, from what I've seen and experienced. I just want to take a few people along with me, to help them along. I'm not going to go out and preach the Gospel. I'm not that kind of person, but there are people who are just beginning to question, to realize what this is, and maybe I can help them. I tell them to just keep on believing that there's more to life than what you can see. I feel terribly excited about life, and hopeful, and happy. I don't have false hope that everything's going to be fine, but I have hope, *and I know it's all right.*

What we observed was a *vibrant* spirituality among these storytellers. For many, their religion had previously been mostly intellectual or social. It was plain that their new spirituality was so real and vital to them precisely because it was based on their own direct experience. During quantum change many, particularly those with epiphanies, experienced themselves in the presence of that which is infinitely great and the nature of which is unspeakably loving. It is the kind of fire that has filled the founders of religions. Over the centuries the adherents of a religion may become distanced, estranged from the fire that gave rise to their traditions. The experience is no longer fresh and firsthand, no longer theirs, except by heritage. Traditions, when divorced from the reasons for their existence, can become stale and empty, their sacredness derived not from the inspiration of meeting the holy through them but merely from the fact that they *are* traditions. Only the hunger remains, never quite sated by going through the traditional motions.

Often quantum change seems to connect or reconnect the person directly with that which transcends them and which unites them with all of humanity and life. Consequently, their spirituality is not isolated, not separate from the rest of their life. Rather, it becomes the lens through which they now perceive all of life.

SELF-ACTUALIZATION

Three schools of thought have dominated the history of clinical psychology. To oversimplify a bit, think of a two-story building with a basement. Psychodynamic theories emphasize the influence of the past, the unconscious foundations, the cellar of human personality. Behavioristic theories occupy the ground level and emphasize the ways in which present behavior interacts with environmental stimuli and reinforcers. The upper floor is occupied by humanistic psychology, the reigning school of American "pop" psychology since the 1960s. Its central emphasis is on the future, on human potential unfettered by the past.

A key concept in humanistic psychology is *self-actualization*, the process of realizing one's own potential and becoming that which one is meant to be. This perspective assumes that a person is not a blank slate but has a unique nature much like the potential found in a seed. Given proper conditions, the seed grows into a particular kind of mature living being. Speaking to health professionals about this natural potential in clients they counsel, Abraham H. Maslow[24] observed: "We already have a start; we already have capacities, talents, direction, missions, callings. The job is, if we are to take this model seriously, to help them to be more perfectly what they already are, to be more full, more actualizing, more realizing in fact what they are in possibility." Some of the quantum changers we spoke with went on to develop new careers as a therapist, a social reformer, a service missionary, and a legislator. One left his longstanding high-tech job and moved to the mountains.

One way to think about what has happened to quantum chang-ers is that they have made a sudden leap forward in self-actualiza-tion. Indeed, many of the attributes that Maslow described as char-acteristic of self-actualized people parallel those reported by quantum changers. They are not self-absorbed, but rather are con-scious of and committed to the world beyond their own skin. They place a high value on honesty, sometimes with painful consequences such as the loss of close friends and relationships. They have a sense of the sacred, and of responsibility not only for themselves, but to others and the world around them. At the same time, pleasing and being approved of by others is of lesser importance. They have a clearer sense of who they are and who they are not. Maslow believed that mystical or "peak" experiences are glimpses or "transient mo-ments of self-actualization,"[25] but that the real thing is the result of a lifelong growth process. Indeed, as described in Chapter 10, many mystical experiences are not life transforming. In quantum change, however—whether of the mystical or insightful type—the person seems to pass through a one-way door, experiencing a sudden large and lasting leap in the process of self-actualization, as though the process had been set for a few moments on fast-forward.

A PROCESS OF CONSOLIDATION

Yet it is also true that the change does not happen all at once. Many of our storytellers emphasized that their experience was not just an event but the beginning of an ongoing process. Although there was a dramatic triggering event, the process of change went on for some time. It was common for them to describe their experience as *still* going on, more than a decade later on average:

> *The effects have lasted totally. As a matter of fact, I would say they're evolving. I don't think they're finished. That's the interesting thing. I don't think that the experience was just that point in time, that five-minute period. I would say that the change is still happen-ing to me, or at least the actual results of that change.*

There was a blending of "it happened" and "it is happening." While some thought that the change had occurred all at once, many described a progression of change after their initial experience. They often understood it as a kind of maturing process as they integrated their new perspective. Sometimes other, smaller experiences followed over the years after the initial quantum change. One woman described it as "a primary earthquake, followed by a series of aftershocks." Transformation did not always happen completely in the twinkling of an eye. Although they had a clear and immediate sense of being permanently changed, some continued for a time in their old ways. The sea captain who wrote "Amazing Grace," for example, was inspired by a transformational experience that happened while he was transporting a shipload of slaves. Yet he continued to make several more slaving voyages before finally redirecting his life. There seems to be a period of consolidation, of integration, after a quantum event:

> *This experience had a transforming effect—I mean, overnight. What had been OK or acceptable was suddenly not acceptable in my life. I burned in the fireplace, almost like a little ritual, my pornographic material, magazines that I had, films that I had. I began reading the Bible. There's a verse in the New Testament which says that you cannot serve God and mammon at the same time. I decided that being gay was not acceptable in the eyes of God. I became what I would call a sunbeam for Jesus. A sunbeam for Jesus is somebody who walks around trying to save everybody else—"Have you found the Lord?"—and talking about God. It was a new experience for me. I did that for about two years and I got wise to myself when I saw another sunbeam who was trying to save me. I'd already been saved. So I kind of cooled it. I decided that whatever I had was a quiet thing; it was an inner thing. If anyone wanted to talk about it, we would talk about it.*
>
> *It affected my nursing in that it gave me a whole new dimension to my work. If there were patients who had cancer, if they had a Bible or the New Testament at their bedside, I felt comfortable sitting down and talking to them about God and about the experience they were going through. It offered a whole new dimension.*
>
> *I still drank for five years after this experience. I was cleaning up my life. I was making amends to people, though nowhere*

near the level of Alcoholics Anonymous. AA gave me something. I
don't think I could have gotten into AA if I had not had that spiritual experience. For me staying sober is a three-part deal: me;
my Higher Power, which is God; and AA. You take away any one
of those three parts and I'll be drunk. For the five years that I
had God before I was in AA, I sat on the bed with a Bible in one
hand and a drink in the other. It was kind of like having a book
but not being able to read. You can look at the pictures and get a
general idea, but once you join AA you learn how to read and all
of it takes on a whole new meaning.

I wasn't looking for what happened to me. That is more than
anybody can ever dream of. I was actively seeking a Higher
Power of some understanding. Some atheists and I had a spiritual
experience once in Vietnam, but that was nothing like this one. If
I believed in a God then, in Nam, it was a God who hated my
guts, or a kind of voodoo God: I'll be good if you don't kill me.
My sunbeam phase was also a voodoo God phase: if you do good
things, then good things will happen to you; if you do bad things,
then you'll get punished. I don't believe now that it happens like
that at all. Things happen, and God can either do something
about it or not do something about it. Whatever He does, He does
for His own reasons, not mine. I can't explain it, really. I don't
share this with everybody I meet. I tried, early on in the first two
years, and I finally came to an acceptance that whatever it was
that happened to me, well, actually there are two words for it:
one is "blessing"—I've been blessed, all right; the other is "miracle." I try to stay away from words like these because they are so
overused by televangelists, but obviously, in a very real sense, it
was a blessing, a miracle. I realize that there are devout people,
religious people who go to church week after week, every Sunday,
all their lives, who have never had an experience like I have had.

It saved my life. It gave meaning to my life. I can't say it
gave purpose to my life yet because I haven't found what my purpose in life is, except to be of use. My sponsor says it's to love
and to serve.

I'm still gay.

I went to many, many churches, essentially trying to recap-
ture the moment that I had in the car that day, trying to find
what I now understand to be spirituality, and I was not finding it
at all. Five years later I walked into AA to find exactly what I

was looking for—to find out I have alcoholism, and to find that the God I believe in is fine. It's my God, of my understanding, and not somebody else's. It's a God that I understand and believe in, and you believe in your God, and that's fine. We're not trying to compare notes. In the New Testament I came across the knowledge that God forgives us. All you have to do is say, "Please forgive me for my sins," and it says right there in the Bible, why God forgives you for your sins. I had trouble with that in my first year or two after this event, to believe that it could be so simple, that God would forgive me. When I finally accepted that, I still wasn't comfortable until one day I was in the shower and I thought, "Wait a minute. Here's your problem. You haven't forgiven yourself. You can't forgive yourself, knowing all you've done. Well, then, what you're saying is you're more powerful than God. If the most powerful being there is can forgive you, then why can't you forgive yourself?" I couldn't answer that one. I had to forgive myself, and it took a while for that to really sink in. I couldn't get it until I came to AA. In five years in AA, I'm still sober with Jesus Christ as my Higher Power. It was a momentous thing that happened to me initially, and also this has been a slow, long, gradual process of growth.

What is it that changes in quantum change? Everything, or at least it seems like everything in the person's inner world has changed: emotions; values; spirituality; sense of self and personal growth; significant relationships; understanding of the past, present, and future. And from the perspective of the recipient, all of it had changed, and continued to change, for the better. This is not at all to say that life became perfect—either immediately or eventually. The desert is still the desert, and yet as in Don Eaton's story (Chapter 11), that which before seemed dry and empty takes on a new light, a new meaning, a kind of perfect imperfection.[26]

17

ARE QUANTUM CHANGES ALWAYS POSITIVE?

Human nature is not compounded wholly of light, but
also abounds in shadows.

—Carl G. Jung[27]

The stories of quantum changers are, in general, remarkably positive, even ecstatic. Nearly all who described to us a quantum change experience said that it had had a dramatically and enduringly beneficial impact on their lives. Writing about peak experiences, Abraham H. Maslow[28] asserted that "the peak experience is only good and desirable, and is never experienced as evil or undesirable. . . . It is reacted to with awe, wonder, amazement, humility and even reverence, exaltation and piety."

Yet we have pondered whether there may be a negative parallel to or form of quantum change. Certainly there are many people who have been devastated by unwanted and unexpected external events, whose lives were forever altered by tragedy. Their experiences were clearly uninvited and often are vividly recalled. Yet the assault of such calamity usually resembles neither the insightful nor the mystical type of quantum change (although Chapter 15 told the unusual story of one catastrophic injury that was accompanied by a deeply positive personal transformation). Such traumatic events usually

144

lack the "aha" sense of insight and the numinous sense of mystical experience. Quantum changes also have a sense of arising from within, or from a mystical source, rather than being a normal reaction to an external event.

Nevertheless, we did encounter a few stories that resembled the quantum changes described in this book in all respects except that their impact was experienced as negative rather than positive. Instead of instilling a sense of peacefulness, they left a pall of doom. In this chapter we relate two examples, one of the insightful type and the other clearly mystical in nature. The first of these happened in the aftermath of a murder-suicide that was mentioned earlier. A teenage girl awoke to discover her mother on the floor, slain by the same gun that her father had used to end his own life. The quantum change experience that she described was not this terrible event itself, however, but a startling realization that occurred one week later.

ORPHANED

I knew that I was an orphan, but I also knew we had a family. We had a grandmother, aunts and uncles, cousins, a whole family like you spend Christmas with and Easter. A week later, after the funeral, I didn't have a family anymore. I was put into foster care. I had grown up with structure, and in the course of a week I had no structure. I had no support. Every aspect of my life from getting up and brushing my teeth, to going to school and church, to knowing who I was, was over. I had nothing but me. There was a judge who decided my life. My grandparents said they were too old to take me. An aunt and uncle took my brother but said that they couldn't handle more than one of us, so since I was adopted they'd take my brother and not me. I was alone.

I remember sitting in my parents' friends' living room—it's like it was yesterday—telling myself that I shouldn't even have a name. I'm not even a person anymore. I'm just a human being, that's it. I have no family. I have no home. I have no life. I have nothing. When I tried to express those feelings to the so-called family services people and the courts over the next two weeks, nobody would listen to me. There were no counselors, no psychiatrists, there was nothing . . . nobody.

So I quit talking. I didn't speak a word for almost a year. I flunked all my school subjects. I didn't socialize. I didn't date, I didn't have anything. Nobody would listen, so I just said "Fine," and I didn't talk. I hardly ate. I felt like life should have been over.

They sent me to a boarding school, and every structure that I knew, every aspect of my life, was different, everything was changed. I got in a lot of trouble with drugs. Downers seemed to really help a lot. Nobody noticed at this boarding school that I was sleeping through classes. I jumped out a third-story window and didn't break anything, but I sure hurt for weeks. Nobody noticed that there was anything wrong with me. I started selling drugs at the school. I progressed quite quickly.

I know exactly when it was that I realized everything was gone. It was right around one o'clock. We were sitting in Arby's restaurant. It's still there. I was with a family who had been friends of my parents. Nobody knew how to talk to me, which—when I look back on it—is very normal. And I was sitting there watching these children interact with their parents, and everybody was having french fries, and they didn't seem to realize I was sitting on the end. It was like I wasn't there, and that's when I realized that I might as well be invisible. I might as well not even be here. I have nobody. I have nobody to put ketchup on my french fries. It was like shock number two, and they were both about the same intensity.

I kept thinking I was sleeping. I kept thinking I was dreaming. It was like I was here and I was physical and I was talking to the judge and talking to the lawyer, and yet I was sitting over at that chair watching this whole thing going on and thinking, "He's not talking to you. You're not really there. You're a nobody. You're not there." It was like I didn't exist. I remember thinking everything seemed to be in slow motion.

The world as I knew it beforehand was friendly, challenging, fun, like a normal teenager's world. After this, life was grim, scary, and a battle. I have some friends who still tell me that I'm very pessimistic and I look at things very darkly. They call me the grim reaper. Before I was very open, and I turned pretty closed to protect myself.

I don't believe in God. I really tried for a long time to get my faith back. Once I started becoming a part of life again, I started going back to mass, observing my holy days, saying my rosary, *and doing all the things that Catholics do. There was a void. I went from one church to another. I went to everything. Nothing. I can't say that I don't believe in God. That's not true. I do believe that there is a Higher Power that did create the sky and the mountains and everything like that, but I don't think that He has any say in our lives. I don't think that if we sit down and pray, this will happen or that will happen. I guess it's kind of sad for my kids, but there's no religion in my house. Before this I believed in God. I said prayers every night. I believed that He would take care of me. It sounds so weird to say this right now. Catholics have this thing called a guardian angel. When I was a kid, my guardian angel took care of me, but at the lowest, worst time in my life, when I needed my guardian angel and God, they were nowhere to be found.*

I have a hard time thinking about the future. I have no re-tirement. None. I've never thought about retirement until the last couple of months. I live not so much for today but for this month. That's what I consider my future. I was talking about this last night because I had this friend in graduate school and he wants me to come down in May. May is like forever. Forget it. I don't make future plans more than just next week. Making this date with you to come here for this visit a week away, that's like about as much as you'll get me to make plans in advance. I just don't. I can't. I cannot. I've never been able to do that, and I don't think I ever will.

*   *   *

The second example does not seem to have been so devastating in the long run but was decidedly a less positive experience than the many other mystical quantum change stories that we heard. A note-worthy difference in its context is that the experience was at least partially drug induced.

DECIDE!

I was born and raised a Catholic. I wouldn't say that I had any unique experiences growing up as a kid. At the time I had my expe-rience I was a student in college, twenty-one or twenty-two years old. I was concentrating on my studies and having a good time like students do.

I had gone with a friend to visit a cousin of mine during spring break. We got there, and she had a girlfriend who was staying with her, maybe a roommate. We just goofed around for a couple days and played tennis and things like that. One night we smoked some dope. They had a unique way of smoking marijuana that involved a large tube that you drew the cigarette smoke into and then somebody would take a hit off of one end. You got a tremendous hit. I took a hit of this thing, and I was immediately higher than a kite. I lay back in the chair and just sat there. I was actually thinking at the time that I was going to try to meld my mind with this friend of mine. I was high, and this was really getting weird. I was thinking we'd communicate without talking or something like that.

That's when this bright light started appearing. The ceiling started getting brighter, and I felt a crushing sensation on my chest. It was like there was a crack in the ceiling and this light started coming through it and getting bigger and brighter. I had been high before and just basically felt silly, but nothing like trying to meld minds with somebody. When that light began to shine on the ceiling and I felt the pressure on the chest, that's when I knew something definitely was weird. I couldn't get out of the chair. At first I was sitting up straight, and it just kind of pushed me back gradually into the chair.

Then all of a sudden, I can't tell you exactly how it occurred, but I started becoming aware of how my actions and inactions, my comments to other people and things I hadn't said to other people at times had affected their lives, basically for the worse. It was amazing. It wasn't big things; it was the little things that were incredible to me: things I had said to someone, and something nice I hadn't said to someone when I had an opportunity to say it. I was seeing only the negative side of what I had done in my life, and all this time the pressure was increasing and I could not get out of that chair. Physically I couldn't have gotten out of that chair if I'd wanted to. I had to sit through this. I wanted to get up and shed it from myself, but I couldn't. I was crushed into that chair. I saw how I must have fouled these people's lives. I knew how these things that I did had affected them. It wasn't a question of yes or no, maybe I did this or maybe I didn't. I had *to accept that it was a fact. All this happened in a flash, in a moment. I really can't tell you how long it was. I'm certain that it happened in one side of the playing of this Moody Blues album, and I'm talking about from when we started smoking until when this thing concluded.*

After that there was a transition. I can't tell you how that transition occurred, but all of a sudden I was shown that everything isn't miserable. There's another side to this coin. I experienced what I would call absolute joy and peace. First, there was this guilt trip thing. This is how you've impacted people, but there's another side to this coin, and that is that you can experience love and peace and joy with these same people. I felt that. It was like a burden lifted, not just the burden of what I'd experienced right then, but a previous burden. It was like a level of joy and peace that I had never known. Now, basically I had never been an unhappy person. As a student I was having a good time in college and getting good grades. I'd never done anything that the world would consider an evil thing, but I had never experienced that kind of joy. The sensation of pressure on my chest was gone.

Then I was made to feel—I had the sensation that I had to choose to accept this joy and peace, that it wasn't a chance I was going to always have, and that I had to accept it or not accept it. I started thinking, "Well, what are the ramifications of this? What does it exactly mean?" I started pacing the room. I can't tell you what the other people were doing at the time. They must have thought I was crackers. Part of the experience of this joy was that people were all in unity, that everybody knew each other completely. In fact, that was part of the joy, that I knew everything you'd done in your life and how your life has affected other people, and that you knew me, completely.

I was pacing the room, thinking, "What does it mean?" It's like I could communicate with something, with this light that was in the ceiling initially. I was asking it, "What does this mean? What does it mean if I accept this?" I wouldn't get an answer, except "You have to decide. Do you want it or don't you?" I started to come up with these excuses as to why I wouldn't want it, basically wrapped around the fact that your life was open, completely open. I knew that was a fact—if I accepted this thing, my life would be completely open—and that was a point of contention. I didn't want it to be, despite the feeling of joy and peace. "Well, what if I just remain like I am, because then I can better communicate with my friends and tell them about this?" I was sort of debating with this thing, this being. I tried to make my case, but I kept having the sensation: "No, you have to decide. Do you want this peace and joy or don't you?" I thought, "Does this mean that I'm going to die? If I accept this, does it mean I'm going to heaven or what? What does it mean? I want an answer to that!" And still it came back: "No, you have to make a decision right now." The sensation was "You have to make a decision, and I'm not giving you any answers. You've seen both sides of this coin, and you have to choose one." None of that was explained to me, I just knew it. Basically it was "You make a decision. You've got the data."

All the time I'm pacing this floor, and after a while I found that I couldn't walk as far in one direction as I could before. When I turned around to walk the other way I found the same thing. I started walking a shorter and shorter line, until finally I got to the middle of the floor and couldn't move. I had to make a decision.

I said, "No, I don't want it."

It was early springtime in the mountains, so it was kind of chilly outside. As soon as I made that decision, I was able to get out of the room. Before that I had boundaries on me. I ran out the door, and I think I left without my jacket on. It was freezing cold, and I was in an absolute paranoid state at that point. I'd gone from that peace and joy to what I've come to think of afterward as an absence of love, the absence of God. I didn't want to speak to anybody or anything. I couldn't communicate. I was frightened, scared to death. I think my friends chased me and made me put my jacket on. I can remember that. I got to the sidewalk, and they made me put my jacket on. I was real freaky, so they just followed me. I don't know where I went or how long this was, but I went all over the city, just out of my gourd. I had a feeling like everybody on the street was just like I was: afraid to talk to each other, hating each other, not wanting to reveal anything about themselves to each other. I remember going down corridors, long corridors, and everything was weird. The corridors were stark and perfectly fit my mood, no colors.

Eventually I made my way back to that room. I'm not sure

how. Maybe these people led me back or something, but eventually I got back into the house, and I was in this paranoid frightened state until the morning. At the end of the night I was able to at least sit still. I was at least at a point where I could stop running. I remember sitting there in that room thinking, "God, am I ever going to be normal again? Am I always going to be paranoid and wacko like this?"

I can't remember if I fell asleep or if it just finally went away. When I woke up the next day, God had basically returned me to sanity.

Afterward I felt like I definitely had been through something real, and it was something I had to think about, consider, act on somehow. This is my own compulsion—I didn't have this Being or whatever compelling me anymore. I felt like I had to figure out what that was all about. I was curious about what had happened, but nobody really wanted to talk about it. I felt different in the sense that I had new knowledge I didn't have before, that there was a good and an evil in the world. I believed in God before the experience, but I don't think I took it that seriously. I believed in God like people "believe in God," if you know what I mean. They're raised that there's a God, so they just believe it. I was fairly certain that this was a religious experience and that God was the Being who was forcing me to make that decision and showing me that there were two sides of the coin from which to choose. I had spiritual awareness that I had never had before. I didn't necessarily see another dimension; I just knew that it was there, for a fact, when I never did before. I felt like I wanted to study. Right after that I read the Bible, completely. I felt that people really do have to make a choice between good and evil eventually. I don't know when it is, whether it's before death, or after, or during.

I think it was an intervention by God in my life, showing me the evil side of life, showing me that even though, as the world sees me, I was a good person, that there was sin in my life, specifically that I'm a sinner and that death is the chasm that exists between me and Him, yet it's a simple thing to bridge that. I always wondered what would have happened if I would have accepted what was offered to me, because that's all it would have taken. I don't have that peace and joy. I feel a lot like I did before really. I don't have any more spiritual insight into other people now than I had before, except that I know what sin is now. I'm a charitable person, where I wasn't before. I mean I give to causes and things. But mostly this is more of an inward experience, a self-examining experience.

I'm a committed Christian now, and I argue biblical principles and things like that. Still, I'm not one to try to force my opinions on other people. I never tried to convert people to Christianity or anything like that. There are a lot of questions left in my mind over this thing, too. It didn't solve a lot. It opened up more questions than it answered. Like I said, I read the Bible from cover to cover, and I continue to read it all the time now. I like to listen to preachers on the radio, and oftentimes the things they say touch a chord of this experience. As long as it's been— twelve years now—I'm still trying to deal with this thing.

I can't tell you why exactly I believe this was a Christian type of experience. In what little I know about Eastern religions, they tell you that there is something positive deep within you that you can bring forward, and that's counter completely to my experience, which was that there's sin in life. It wasn't impressed on me that this was "sin," but it definitely was not good. I came to call it sin afterward, but this Being or this thing that I was sort of communicating with didn't say that this is sin in life and you need to get your act together. I knew what it was. That's why I did study different religions for a while, and my conclusion is that this was more of a Christian-based experience than anything else. It made me aware that sin is such a subtle thing that you just can't give it up. That was something that I wasn't aware of before. It woke me up that I'd better reconsider my life—I'd better delve into the spiritual side of things as well as the intellectual, which is my current pursuit.

*   *   *

These stories, when compared with those in prior chapters, evoke a rather different response in the listener. We were deeply saddened by the first story of a gregarious, fun-loving teenager robbed by tragedy of her optimism, her joy, and her faith. Was it a quantum change? Certainly the magnitude of effect is similar, and she vividly remembered the two moments when it hit, the insight that changed her life. Her story might be explained away as an example of posttraumatic stress disorder, and victimization can surely trigger a devastating personal transformation. Trauma can itself leave a person demoralized, hypervigilant, hopeless, and pervasively helpless. Merely to give her experience a diagnostic name, however, neither explains it nor renders it automatically different from quantum change. The topography of this experience resembles in many ways the process of quantum change described in earlier chapters, except in photographic negative.

Perhaps trauma has the potential to produce quantum change that can be either positive or negative in form. Some of the quantum changes that people experienced as profoundly benevolent arose in the midst of traumatic events: a broken neck (Chapter 15), a tortuous abortion (Chapter 10), a family crisis (Chapter 3). Another man described the following negative experience that occurred when his young sister was hospitalized for treatment of schizophrenia:

> *She decided that God was talking to her, telling her to do specific things like burn down our house, or lie naked underneath a car in a parking lot at 3 o'clock in the morning in subzero weather. They locked her up—straitjacket, the whole nine yards—and I went up and visited her and I decided then and there that if this was God, I didn't want to have anything to do with him. I think that's when I really started going downhill physically and emotionally and spiritually, and I really slid into a skid row kind of alcoholism, drinking all day long, every day, because nothing mattered.*

If indeed these are examples of the same phenomenon in destructive form, a deeper understanding of quantum change might lead to a better grasp of how people can be damaged by trauma, and perhaps to better ways for helping them.

The above story of a drug-related experience is fascinating for the further questions that it raises. While the other examples in this chapter resemble the insight type of quantum change, "Decide!" is clearly an epiphany. It suggests an element of *choice* in quantum change, the necessity of openness to the experience. Perhaps that element was a drug-induced aberration, or perhaps the drug state somehow sharpened awareness of a choice component that is normally less salient. Quantum changers sometimes say that their experience forced them to make a choice, and some indeed choose an entirely new lifestyle as a result of their experience. Usually this choice is experienced as warm and welcome, rather than the fearsome demand placed on this young man. It is a poignant story, full of pathos. As readers, we identify and ask ourselves, "What would I have done?" One cannot but wonder whether the storyteller would get a second chance. The hallmarks of a mystical quantum change are clearly there, but somehow reshaped (perhaps by the drug) into a terrifying and intimidating experience. He is left, in the end of the story, at the beginning of a spiritual quest.

This story also highlights the interesting overlap of quantum change and drug-induced mystical experiences. In a twenty-five-year follow-up study of seven seminary students who had participated in a study of psilocybin-induced mystical experiences, participants had vivid recall of the event and reported some enduring beneficial effects. There are clear similarities between these psilocybin-induced states and the reports of drug-free quantum change experiences. What is strikingly different from the reports of quantum changers is the frequency and intensity of emotionally aversive experiences (terror, paranoia, death) during the drug induced state. The participants had also had mystical experiences that were not drug induced, and they were able to compare them. "The non-drug experiences were composed primarily of peaceful, beautiful moments experienced with ease while the drug experiences tended to include moments of great fear, agony and self-doubt."[29]

What these two stories together suggest is that there are specific events that can trigger personal transformation that is at least similar to quantum change, and that is not always benevolent in nature. Traumatic events and drug-induced states are two obvious candidates. It is tempting for us to say that these are somehow "artificial" or "exogenous" quantum changes, arising in reaction to an external physical agent. Yet the line is not so clear, and it is circular to classify quantum changes as natural or artificial based on the benevolence of outcome. These stories leave open the possibility that at least under some conditions, an experience of (or like) quantum change can be enduringly detrimental or disabling. In these shadows may lie important clues for understanding the nature of quantum change.

18

WHAT HAPPENED?

The end of one thing is the beginning of another. I am
a pilgrim again.
    —YUICHIRO MIURA, *The Man Who Skied Down Everest*[30]

We set out on this journey in order to understand quantum change. We believed, and still believe, that these stories contain the seeds of a powerful form of change, with great potential for healing. The personal accounts in themselves are fascinating and mysterious, but we wanted more. If quantum change stories do offer clues to a qualitatively different kind of healing that happens in human lives, what hope do they offer to those still struggling with some demon or heavy burden? How might the gift of these stories help to shine new light into other tragedies? For us as psychologists, that was a wish always lurking beneath the surface of our passion for these stories. We set out not just to hear and tell stories but to *understand* quantum change in the hope that such understanding might contribute to means for healing.

A decade later we have a reasonably good description of the phenomenon and full confidence that sudden, profound and enduring positive changes can and do occur in the lives of real people. Lives are transformed utterly and permanently, as utter darkness suddenly gives way to a joyful dawn that had not even been imagined. It happens.

Yet description is far from understanding. An aboriginal bush-man could describe an airliner passing overhead without any un-derstanding of jet propulsion or aerodynamics. Great minds have wrestled with this mystery before and settled for description. Wil-liam James concluded: "Now if you ask of psychology just *how* . . . and *why* aims that were peripheral became at a certain moment central, psychology has to reply that although she can give a gen-eral description of what happens, she is unable in a given case to account accurately for all the single forces at work."[31] Psychologi-cal theories are reasonably good at explaining the changes that oc-cur in *discrete* behavior and cognition (such as a belief, a memory, a phobia, or the drinking of alcohol), but we know of nothing in behavioral science that adequately describes (let alone explains) the sudden, sweeping, and permanent transformations of quantum change. One can imagine, in hindsight, that some quantum changes were the culmination of a developmental process, but this is not an adequate explanation of when, how, and why they occur. Although some behaviorists have acknowledged and even docu-mented the phenomenon of transformational change,[32] none has offered a satisfactory explanation.

So having described quantum change, what can we say about how and why it happens? It is a daunting task, presuming to push past the point where scholars like William James have thrown in the towel. Certainly it would be pretentious for us to claim we have found the secret of quantum change. Yet we have had a privileged opportunity to hear firsthand so many personal accounts, and a cen-tury of psychology has accumulated since James's classic volume, af-fording us a variety of lenses through which to view the phenome-non. We feel obliged not to settle for a portrait, engaging though it be. In the interest of moving past description, we offer in this chap-ter not one but five perspectives on how and why quantum change may occur, based on our research thus far. We have termed them as follows:

1. Breaking point
2. Deep discrepancy
3. Personal maturation
4. Particular person
5. Sacred encounter

1. BREAKING POINT

One way of explaining quantum change experiences is that they represent a *kairos*, a turning point in the life journey where major change simply must occur because the person is unable or unwilling to continue in his or her present course. It is a point of desperation, a breaking point where "something has to give"—and it does. Remember the young babysitter so paralyzed by fear that she could only spin in circles in the middle of the room lest someone sneak up behind her (Chapter 3). It is not hard to imagine that the very intensity of her terror forced her to snap out of this miasma of fear. Other storytellers had spiraled downward into such desperation that they could only turn for help to something greater and wiser than themselves. They reached the end of their rope, and then it snapped.

The result is a new, dramatically reorganized identity. One might draw an analogy here to the development of multiple personality disorder, where early trauma is so great that one's identity is segmented, dissociated into separate parts. In quantum change, it is almost the opposite process. Strained and separate aspects of identity are reordered in one brilliant moment. The deck is reshuffled. The pieces are moved around, and at some level the person suddenly sees how they can be rearranged into a new picture of self. The crisis is resolved by that person becoming someone new. It happens not as a controlled and conscious decision but in a sudden flash that the person experiences as not of his or her own doing. The reorganization happens almost automatically, without intention or planning.

The storyteller of "A Mirror and Two Roses" (Chapter 7) clearly describes his pre-quantum-change life as reaching such a breaking point: "I guess you would say I hit rock bottom. I had a lack of confidence, really poor self-image. I was very unhappy, very depressed. I didn't like myself. I didn't like other people." He was living "in a hellhole" and drinking heavily; then suddenly he was transformed. The stories of Chapter 17 suggest that such reorganization can also occur in negative as well as positive ways. The new picture of identity and reality can come into focus in photographic negative rather than positive. Unlike in multiple personality disorder, however, the new identity (be it positive or negative) is stable. One can imagine a sudden adult trauma as a catalyst for such reconceptualization of self. Indeed, the stories in this volume illustrate that traumatic events can be associated with either profoundly positive (Chapter 15) or deeply negative reorganization (Chapter 17).

If the new vision of self and reality arises from within the person, then it must be a composite of images that were already available to the person. The resolution breaks upon consciousness with great force, but it is constituted from building-block resources that were already present. In this regard, other people may play a key role in determining the possible selves from which a new identity is forged. Parents, friends, teachers, healers, clergy, social groups— all may suggest images of how one *can* be, the possible selves from which one may choose when a *kairos* is reached. In some cases, a person who is immediately present at the time of the quantum change (like the guru in "Taking the AA Train," Chapter 6) may have a substantial influence on the reconceptualized self.

Some social reference groups also offer strong guidance for how identity can or should be reshaped. Alcoholics Anonymous (AA) centers on the "twelve steps" as a way of living, and the first-hand account of their author, Bill Wilson, is unambiguously a quantum change story. There are many such stories in AA. Many religious organizations provide clear prescriptions and proscriptions for living that can provide a new model after a conversion experience. The phenomenon of religious conversion represents, as an ideal at least, a radical and permanent reorganization of identity. Some therapeutic and commercial "movements," such as est (Erhard Seminars Training) and its more recent born-again forms, are designed specifically to trigger a quantum change and offer a particular vision of the good life to which one should be reborn. Unfortunately, there is no reliable research evidence for the efficacy of such approaches.

Even if methods for reliably inducing quantum change were identified, there would be vexing ethical issues involved in providing the template to which identity should be reshaped, particularly when such reformation efforts are implemented during a time of personal crisis and vulnerability. Yet it is unavoidable, at least within the psychological breaking point and reintegration view, that the foundation stones for a post-quantum-change identity are provided by one's history and relationships.

2. DEEP DISCREPANCY

If it is a breaking point, a peak crisis that triggers quantum change, then what about those individuals who were not in any obvious crisis or personal pain at the time of transformation? What about the Scrooges who, from their pre-quantum-change perspective, were perfectly content, thank you, and did not desire change? One can press the breaking-point model by asserting that "really" they were coming apart, but there is nothing more than speculation to support this view within some of the stories we heard. Such speculation stretches people in Procrustean fashion to fit a breaking-point model. Without the means to test the assertion directly, it is circular to argue that an apparently contented person who underwent a quantum change had, in fact, been in crisis.

Perhaps, though, there is some hidden observer within each person that perceives a crisis below conscious awareness and calls for a sudden course correction in spite of conscious better judgment. The idea of unconscious conflict erupting into behavior change has been central to psychodynamic theories since the early writings of Sigmund Freud. Is it possible that a profound conflict or discrepancy has been building below awareness for some time and finally erupts in a quantum change that the person experiences as not of his or her own doing? Perhaps a consciously experienced crisis or breaking point is just one form of a broader phenomenon that triggers transformation. Several of the stories told earlier in this book (consider Chapters 5, 6, and 13) describe people who were not consciously in crisis and at a breaking point, yet who were at some level aware of deep discrepancies between where they were and where they could be.

The danger of circular reasoning is noteworthy here, but there is well-substantiated psychological theory from which this possible explanation can be extrapolated. It is a longstanding observation in psychology that at least two different processes of change seem to operate in human life. As discussed in Chapter 1, William James differentiated the gradual "educational" variety of change from sudden transformation. The study of cognition has revealed two distinct systems of memory. Learning can occur by gradual approximations or by a sudden "aha" insight. Human behavior change has been described as occurring via two general systems: *automatic* processes that operate mostly below conscious awareness, and *controlled* processes that are more effortful.

The general process by which we humans change in response to the world around (and within) us has been called *self-regulation*.[33] At both conscious and unconscious levels, we are constantly comparing what we perceive with how we think things ought to be. In driving, for example, we proceed on down the road as long as conditions seem normal. When something out of the ordinary happens, however—such as an object moving into our field of vision on a collision course—we take action: attend closely, slow down or speed up, or perhaps swerve or change course. Driving is a largely unconscious process of scanning for anything "out of the ordinary"— anything that doesn't match our sense of safety and normality.

In the same way, we tend to keep on moving down the same path in our lives until something tells us that a change is needed— that there is a significant discrepancy between how things are and how we want them to be. Such discrepancies tend to trigger a change in behavior, and the change can be either gradual or sudden.[34] The usual route of change is that people operate on automatic pilot until they run into signals that something is wrong.

With something as simple (yet complex) as driving down a city street, one operates the vehicle without much conscious effort. It is not uncommon to arrive at a destination without having paid much attention to the process of getting there. When one is first learning to drive, these same skills are quite self-consciously controlled, but as they become familiar and routine they become automatic processes. It is only when one perceives something out of the ordinary that the process becomes more aware and planfully controlled.

The same thing occurs in larger areas of life. People often continue on with a habit—be it drinking alcohol, overworking, or criticizing others—until something appears on the radar screen to tell them that they are on a collision course. It might be something dramatic, like an arrest or a heart attack. Sometimes (as in Chapter 7, "A Mirror and Two Roses") it can be as simple as looking in a mirror or having a friend say, "You're fat." Ordinarily this wake-up call engages a conscious process of searching for alternatives: "What can I do to change?" Having been driving along on automatic pilot, the person now consciously turns the wheel to head off in a new direction. Such change is usually experienced as willful, intentional, and self-regulated.

Part of the fascination of quantum change is that this ordinary process is turned upside down. The enduring charm of *A Christmas Carol* is not that Scrooge saw the error of his ways and consciously pulled himself up by his own bootstraps. Old Scrooge, in fact, saw nothing wrong with his controlled way of life. Instead, his boots were pulled out from under him and for a night he went tumbling out of control. When he again landed on his feet on Christmas morning, he was a changed man not through his own effort and merit but by an uninvited and unmerited spiritual intervention. Quantum change is like that. Rather than the automatic processes giving way to controlled change, it is the other way around. Something just snaps. People going along in their usual consciously controlled way of life find themselves abruptly changed. It's a bit like a "mental breakdown" in reverse. The result can be a profoundly positive rebuilding, a rebirth, a new way of seeing and being. One man, whose father had struggled with alcoholism, characterized his pre-quantum-change personality as perfectionistic and compulsive, with a seething hostility that would erupt in rage at home or behind the wheel of his car. Looking back on his insightful quantum change, he observed:

> *I realized that I was now identifying with what it is to be a real human being instead of with stereotypical attributes of what a person should be. I remember saying to myself, before all this happened, that it's important to be friendly, gentle, caring, helpful—all those things—but I was intellectualizing it all. With the change, it seems like now I feel it inside. It's amazing to go from thinking about your feelings to actually feeling your feelings. Somehow or other I got in touch with that, and as I did, the walls started to break down and it all started to come in on me.*

If self-regulatory course adjustments happen at a molecular behavioral level, they may also occur on a wider scale. Carl R. Rogers[35] wrote of discrepancies at the level of the self: between the actual self (who I am) and the ideal self (who I ought to or would like to be). Disturbances of self-concept are also reflected in the preceding stories. The storyteller of "Something Like a Star" (Chapter 12) expressed what he was experiencing prior to his quantum change: "about being a failure financially, about hurting my children, about life being absolutely no fun anymore. I just felt like there was no reason to live." In Chapter 7, "A Mirror and Two Roses," the storyteller said this of his pre-quantum-change state: "I had a lack of confidence, really poor self-image. I was very unhappy, very depressed. I didn't like myself. I didn't like other people."

Psychologist Roy F. Baumeister[36] described a process of "the crystallization of discontent" that triggers change. He characterized this process as

> the forming of associative links among a multitude of unpleasant, unsatisfactory, and otherwise negative features of one's current life situation. Prior to a crystallization of discontent, a person may have many complaints and misgivings . . . but these remain separate from each other. The crystallization brings them together into a coherent body. . . . The subjective impact can be enormous, because a large mass of negative features may be enough to undermine a person's commitment to a role, relationship, or involvement.

Such discontent can be at the level of a single behavior such as smoking or drinking (as in "On the Island" in Chapter 4) or a relationship (such as the marriage in "Awakening," Chapter 8), but it can also occur at an existential level—a dissatisfaction with one's life and person in general. Such was the case for the woman contemplating suicide (in Chapter 3), and perhaps with the high-tension pre-quantum-change lifestyle described in "A Voice in the Fireplace" (Chapter 13).

What is it that triggers such a major reorganization? Many psychological theories posit that change occurs in response to deep discrepancies or conflicts that arise within the person. Milton Rokeach[37] introduced a theory of personality that we find particularly helpful in making sense of sudden reorganizations of character. He conceptualized personality as organized in a series of levels that might be thought of as concentric circles (see the accompanying diagram). At the most shallow or peripheral level are the person's moment-to-moment thoughts, feelings, and actions. Underlying these are countless specific beliefs that tend to shift with experience. Beliefs, in turn, are organized around broader attitudes, which number in the thousands for a given individual.

Behind attitudes and more central to personality are our values, which are the standards we use to evaluate ourselves and others. According to Rokeach, these are of two types. One's *instrumental* values

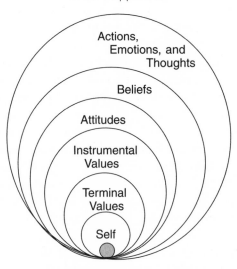

Rokeach's Model of Personality

number a few dozen and represent general ways and means of being in the world: cooperating, forgiving, ambitious, obedient, responsible. Still more central are "a few handfuls" of *terminal* values, the primary ends toward which one's life is directed; some examples of these include personal comfort and security, world peace, pleasure, freedom, and God's will. Some values are more important or central to the individual than others, so that terminal values (ends) are themselves organized in hierarchies, and means (instrumental values) may subserve particular ends. Thus there can be entire systems of interrelated behaviors, functionally linked to clusters of beliefs and attitudes, which in turn are related to underlying instrumental and terminal values.

Finally, most central of all, is the individual's sense of self. This includes describable attributes of self-concept (who I am), as well as that experienced core of identity that persists throughout life—the deepest part of oneself that is somehow the same across all the years and experiences of personal growth or decline. It is the "I" in "I know" or "I am not satisfied with myself." From some perspectives it might be called the soul or spirit of the person.

Now, how does this organization of personality relate to change? The level at which an event occurs affects the breadth and permanence of change. The more central the level at which a change occurs, the more enduring and far reaching its effects are likely to be. Changing a specific *behavior* or *thought* is unlikely to generalize much to the overall personality, and the change may not even endure unless it is backed up by deeper shifts. Changing a specific *belief* (such as the perceived motivation for another person's specific action) may change a few related thoughts and behaviors toward that person. Something that affects one's overall *attitude* about the person, however, may affect a number of beliefs about that person and a larger array of related thoughts, feelings, and actions.

It follows from this that anything as sweeping and enduring as quantum change would have to emanate from shifts at the most central levels of organization. Among others, the storytellers of "Awakening" (Chapter 8) and "Something Like a Star" (Chapter 12) described a comprehensive transformation of their beliefs, attitudes, and values. Such broad changes, Rokeach believed, arise from contradictions involving terminal values and self-concept. If something more peripheral (like a behavior or a belief) comes into conflict with a deeper value, the more peripheral element is likely to change. People who suddenly stop smoking, drinking, or using illicit drugs, for example, may do so when something makes it clear that their drug use is endangering that which they hold dear, a strong value. Values can also come into conflict with one another and with the person's core identity. Change is instigated particularly when a contradiction has implications for self-concept, creating a crisis of self-dissatisfaction. This is evident in the story, "Something Like a Star" (Chapter 12), where it was in part the realization of hurting his children that precipitated the storyteller's abstinence from alcohol. Drinking came into conflict with his love for his children, and drinking lost. Abstinence, in turn, heightened his discontent with much broader aspects of his life. With a growing sense of self-dislike and helplessness, he looked beyond himself for help and found it.

How does all this help make sense of quantum change? It surely is consistent with the report of our participants that changes occurred at many levels and particularly that there were sudden major shifts in what they *valued*. The common report that "*I* changed" (not that "things" or "things about me" changed) suggests involvement all the way to the level of self-conception. A high level of self-dissatisfaction is apparent in many of the stories (see Chapter 3), although for some the self-discontent itself arose suddenly and (as in Scrooge's case) represented a major shift from prior self-conception. The man who went on retreat "At Pecos" (Chapter 14) was not consciously aware of discontent at the time: "I didn't have any particular ideas about what to expect. I wasn't looking for anything in particular; just wanted to have some quiet time, something like that." And yet he went to a monastery searching for *something*, he knew not what.

Quantum changers are not always conscious of major discrepancies in their lives prior to their transformation. Of course, powerful experiences erupting from the unconscious realm are nothing new in psychodynamic theory. Although much theorizing has been focused on pathological products of the unconscious, many ordinary psychological processes (such as perception, learning, and memory) operate below as well as within conscious levels of awareness. Perhaps quantum change is some sort of adjustment or problem-solving process that goes on at a subconscious level, presenting its results only as a finished product. This is consistent with the experience that the quantum change was "not me"—that the person was not the agent of his or her own transformation.

An everyday example is found in the struggle to remember a name or solve a problem. It is a common experience that when conscious effort fails, the answer will pop into awareness later, after a period of rest or focusing on other tasks. "It will come to me later," one says. Some people, after a period of intense concentration, intentionally put the problem on the unconscious back burner with instruction for a solution to be found by incubation. Then later, at a time when the person is "not even thinking about it," there comes the "aha"—in the shower, in a dream or daydream, or driving down the road. Sometimes the solution has to do with an entirely new way of perceiving the problem.

In many respects, quantum changes resemble this kind of incubation process. To be sure, the new perception reorganizes broad aspects of the person and not just a single behavior or problem. Quantum changes do "come to" the person from outside of awareness, but they do so with a peculiar forcefulness. Perhaps quantum changes are products of deep levels of incubation that erupt once a new solution is prepared. Faced with an intolerable level of distress or growing inner discrepancies, the person may work out a synthesis at a subconscious (or, some might say, superconscious[38]) level. The resolution, a reorganization of reality perception, is then admitted to consciousness, where it seems to come "out of nowhere" but is understandably recognized as deeply right or true. Again, to say that the mechanism is unconscious does not explain it but only describes the fact that the work that led up to it is not within the conscious awareness of the individual who experiences it. The person cannot say how it happened, because it just seemed to appear from nowhere.

3. PERSONAL MATURATION

Thinking of quantum change as an incubated solution to personal conflict does not really account for its major significance as a milestone—a unique transforming experience in the person's life. Quantum changers look back on their event as a single turning point, a new beginning in their lives. If it were an unconscious way of working out inner discrepancies, one might expect it to be a repeated experience and perhaps to be given less ultimate importance. Although some people do have several experiences of this kind, they tend to understand them as part of the *same* process that began with the first experience. The first event is qualitatively different from prior experience, sending the person through a one-way door and setting in motion an ongoing and accelerated process of transformation.

Neither do the preceding explanations account for the striking consistency of both content and process that we have observed across quantum change experiences, a topic to which we return in our final chapter. How does it happen that people come from so many different starting points to such similar destinations?

One way to make sense of this is to think of quantum change as a maturational phenomenon. Jean Piaget identified successive, qualitatively distinct steps in cognitive development. A child at the preoperational level of development (roughly ages two to seven) can use language but simply cannot comprehend the relational and planful thinking of the concrete operations stage (roughly ages seven to eleven), let alone the way in which adults (at the formal operations stage) use symbols and abstraction to perceive reality. Lawrence Kohlberg[39] identified parallel stages of moral development, moving from external to internal control. Development begins at a pre-moral stage (behaving to get rewards and avoid punishment) and progresses to a principled set of morals and values that guide behavior, followed because they are perceived to be the right way to live. Again, a person at the pre-moral stage of development would simply not comprehend the principled governance of behavior. From Kohlberg's moral stages, James W. Fowler[40] extrapolated levels of personal faith development, progressing from the simple stages of faith in childhood to a rarely achieved universalizing level characterized by nondogmatic humility, a relative lack of self-concern, and a love for all humanity that is grounded in a profound sense of unity and spiritual interconnectedness. In each of these theories, not everyone reaches the higher stages of development. Some spend their adult lives quite happily at a more simple or concrete level.

Quantum change is often experienced as a kind of personal integration, a consolidation of wholeness and identity. The similarity of quantum change stories to Kohlberg's "universalizing" level is striking. Where there was once discord and confusion, there is a sense of peaceful acceptance and integrity. Quantum changers are disinclined to be dogmatic and frequently report a sense of profound unity with all of humanity or nature. This does not always happen all at once, but there is definitely a discrete jump, a perceptual shift at the point of a quantum change experience. It is possible that quantum change represents a developmental jump, or even a poorly understood advanced level of maturation that is reached by some of us.

Humanistic and existential theorists in particular have written of such nirvana-like farther reaches of human potential, describing processes of self-actualization, peak experience, higher consciousness, and integration. In studying people who had had peak experiences, Maslow[41] initially concluded that they were largely the result of an evolved form of consciousness that is found in highly developed, self-actualized people, although he did acknowledge the "occasional peak experiences of average people." Our experience is quite different. Although we do regard quantum change to be a higher form of consciousness, its experience does not seem to be at all restricted to extraordinary, fully developed human beings. It comes instead, unexpected and uninvited, in the midst of ordinariness or in the depth of despair, and without apparent regard for degree of self-actualization. It was such peak experiences, in fact, that caused Maslow to reevaluate his conception of self-actualization not as "a kind of all-or-none pantheon into which some rare people enter at the age of 60," but as something that can come in "an episode or a spurt" at any time in a person's life.[42] Such a maturational spurt is illustrated in "Taking the AA Train" (Chapter 6) and "Ripples" (Chapter 9).

There is again a parallel here to the phenomenon of religious conversion. Conversion is often confused with religious membership, self-identification, adherence, or affiliation. In this sense, an individual is sometimes described as "converting" to a particular religion. Yet most faith traditions describe true conversion as an inner transformation of the heart, of consciousness.[43] It is understood as an important and deeper process of spiritual development that may not occur until after many years of disciplined practice. For many—perhaps most—adherents of a religion, it may never occur at all in a lifetime. Like quantum change, such transformations are often described as being born through a time of pain or from the inner conflict of opposites. Though the entry process, like birth, may be a painful one, its fruits are characterized as profoundly healing. Longstanding members of AA often express gratitude for the profoundly painful experiences of their alcoholism, without which they might never have found their way to spiritual serenity.

Perhaps quantum change, then, represents a maturational event, one that transports the individual to a higher level of human consciousness. We hasten to add here that none of those who told us their stories bragged about their experience as a badge of achievement, as an attainment of personal endeavor. As described earlier, the most common perception of quantum changers seems to be a grateful sense of giftedness, combined with a humility that pretends no unique qualifications, deservingness, or entitlement. Neither did we find any sense of superiority—that having had such an experience raised them to a better class of humanity. To the contrary, the common experience was that of oneness with all humanity.

Quantum change often results in a profoundly different sense of meaning in life, and it may come especially to those who search for their meaning or purpose. Though sober for fourteen years, the woman hit by the AA train (Chapter 6) was aware of something missing in her work with other alcoholics. The seeker at Pecos (Chapter 14) said of his pre-quantum-change years, "We were looking for the great answer—you know, what life is all about." In all of these, there is a sense of sudden maturation after a period of seeking. Perhaps it is particularly those who seek deeper meaning who find—or are found by—quantum change.

4. PARTICULAR PERSON

Yet another way of explaining quantum change (as well as the consistencies in such experiences) is to say that it only happens to certain kinds of people, and thereby tells us something about the individuals themselves. Perhaps those who experience quantum change possess particular characteristics or life patterns that set them apart and make such experiences uniquely accessible.

What attributes might predispose to the kind of change we have described? A century ago, William James speculated that transformational changes are more likely to occur in people with an "active subliminal self" who seem to have more ready access to the unconscious. He specified three attributes in this regard that may converge to increase the likelihood of sudden transformations: emotional sensitivity, suggestibility (such as hypnotic susceptibility), and a "tendency to automatisms."[44] By the last, he referred to a variety of experiences that from the person's perspective arise from an unknown source. As examples he named unaccountable impulses or inhibitions to act, automatic writing or speech, and ideas that seem to appear out of nowhere. (This is nicely illustrated in "A Mirror and Two Roses," Chapter 7, and by the young seeker on Redondo Beach in Chapter 10.)

The Intuitive Person

In several ways, the experiences described by quantum changers, as well as the attributes highlighted by William James, resemble what Carl G. Jung called the intuitive process of "knowing by the unconscious." Within Jung's theory of personality, this is one normal style of perception.

Its opposite is the sensing style, which involves a preference for relying on information collected step by step through the physical senses. Sensing-type people attend to and trust factual experience, the witness of their five senses. If you ask them how they know something, their reply would probably be admissible in court. Intuitive types have a harder time explaining how they know, because they tend to rely on a "sixth sense." Their natural mode of perception is to see patterns, meanings, and symbols. When they "know" something they may be quite correct, but often they can't point to sensory evidence by which they reached their knowledge. They make jumps that mystify a sensing-type person, who insists, "You can't know that!" One quantum changer described it this way:

> *I tend to learn differently from most of my peers and have since kindergarten, so I was an outcast in school until I got to graduate school, where everybody was doing it my way and I was the one who was making the As instead of the Cs. It's that global thinking versus step-by-step-by-step logic. That's the way my life goes. I never ever get it step-by-step-by-step.*

Both ways of knowing have their advantages and disadvantages, and both modes, in Jung's view, are accessible to everyone. Human differences are in the extent to which we prefer, trust, and rely upon our senses or our intuition to perceive reality.

Several of our quantum changers described this intuitive style as their normal mode of functioning. Any Jungian would recognize this description from a participant in our study:

> *It's like a thought just runs through my mind that makes sense, just like a ticker tape. When something has been bothering me for a long time, it's like I've been looking for a piece of the puzzle. Maybe it's just the last piece in the puzzle that I didn't even know I was working on, and it just clicks into place. I think global; instead of building up to it through a-b-c-d, it's like "There it is," and then you go back and figure out why it makes sense.*

This pattern of suddenly "getting it" is common in quantum change. There are clear examples in insightful quantum change stories: a woman "Awakening" from a hazy identity (Chapter 8), a father's recollections of "The Flood" (Chapter 4), and the sudden emotional "Boom" of seeing a new reality (Chapter 5).

Could it be that quantum changers are intuitive types who are just having a larger version of their usual mode of perception? Among the questionnaires that were completed by participants in our study was the Myers–Briggs Type Indicator.[45] Based on Jungian theory, it measures personality preferences including the sensing–intuitive dimension. We included it precisely because we guessed that it might identify those who are particularly prone to quantum change. Indeed, intuitive types were overrepresented in our sample relative to their minority status among U.S. adults. They constituted seventy-nine percent of those with insightful quantum change experiences and sixty percent of those with mystical quantum change experiences. It could be, of course, that intuitive people were just more likely to come forward to tell their story, being more comfortable with this way of knowing. It is also important to recall that we were talking to butterflies and not caterpillars. With an average of eleven years transpired since the experience, it could be that this personality trait is one of the things altered by quantum change. We do happen to have pre-quantum-change profiles for two storytellers, and both were strongly intuitive types beforehand.

What we *can* conclude, however, is that quantum change is not a phenomenon that happens *only* to intuitive people. Some of the stories were recounted by people who, by their self-description as well as their testing, were unambiguously sensing types. Within Jung's theory, the intuitive process is available to all individuals and can erupt with particular power in a sensing-type person, especially during the second half of life, when people begin to explore their less developed side and questions of meaning begin to emerge. While quantum changes do resemble Jung's description of intuitive/ unconscious knowing, to "explain" them in this way is merely to exchange one description for another. Furthermore, even intuitive types who told us their stories had experienced their quantum change as distinctly different from their ordinary way of knowing, if only by an order of magnitude.

Special Realities

Many of those who told us their stories had led lives that would be judged by social standards to be rather normal. There was nothing out of the ordinary about them, beyond the uniqueness of every human being. Others had suffered a variety of what are commonly termed mental illnesses. A number had been caught in the grip of alcohol and drug dependence. Some had been deeply depressed. One man had his life-changing insight during what he, in retrospect, recognized as a manic episode before his bipolar disorder had been diagnosed and treated. A number of them had suffered posttraumatic effects of childhood physical and sexual abuse. A few had ongoing struggles with what would be diagnosed as psychoses.

Is there a relationship between quantum change and mental disorders? First, and emphatically, we must say that it is vital not to confuse the two. Quantum change clearly happens to ordinary as well as extraordinary people. Mystical experiences have a very long history, and if viewed out of context can be mistaken for mental disorder. This is, perhaps, one reason why those who have experienced quantum changes so often remain silent about them. Such experiences, besides being difficult to communicate, may make other people uneasy. They challenge comfortable assumptions about the limits of reality. A common thread running through the stories is that after such an experience, people often view the material world as merely a small part of a much greater reality, and a relatively unimportant part at that. This insight does not send them into monastic withdrawal from society. To the contrary, it often inspires their devotion of significant time to compassionate service for others. Nevertheless, to reject materialism (in the philosophic as well as hedonistic sense) is to challenge the very assumptions on which a consumer society is based. An easy response to these disquieting stories, then, is to dismiss them as at least temporary madness. Sadly, some who have had such experiences ultimately accept this explanation themselves.

It is possible, however, that people who experience out-of-the-ordinary realities by virtue of what is now diagnosed as mental disorder do have easier access to quantum changes. Attend almost any meeting of AA and you can meet someone who thanks God for being an alcoholic. "Had I not been alcoholic," such people often say, "I might never have found my way into the wonderful spiritual life that I have now. Without alcoholism, I could easily have wasted my entire life." This boggles the mind of one who has not been there. People think they must mean that suffering is good because "it feels so good when it stops," or confuse the message with the cliche, "I complained that I had no shoes until I met a person who had no feet." Rather, what they usually mean is that the alcoholism *itself* was a vital part of their new understanding. Perhaps those whose sense of reality has already been torn away from the "normal" are better prepared to receive whatever it is that quantum change has to offer.[46] Even if one accepts a wholly biological explanation of mental disorders, there is no reason to reject as invalid the quantum changes experienced by people with such disorders, any more than one would dismiss a story because the person had cancer or heart disease. There is much to learn from people whose sense of reality differs from our own.

It is also possible that certain life experiences open a person to the possibility of quantum change. Profound loss is a theme that is evident in a number of these stories. Prolonged distress also recurs as a theme. Such experiences may open a channel of sensitivity or compassion that makes quantum change more accessible.

5. SACRED ENCOUNTER

Our exploration of possible explanations for quantum change would be incomplete if we failed to discuss this final one, which is how a majority of our participants understood what had happened to them. All of the hypotheses discussed above are feasible even if one assumes that material reality is all there is. In these views, the quantum change experience arises somehow within the person's skin, from his or her personality dynamics and brain chemistry. Most adults, however, are not materialists in this sense. They do not believe that the material world is all that exists. Belief in the existence of an unseen spiritual dimension has been normative throughout recorded history, and in the United States more than ninety percent of adults profess belief in its reality, be it in the form of a God, or an afterlife, or other things spiritual that transcend material existence. Here, by definition, we depart from what is directly observable at present, although subjective accounts of spiritual experiences have long been the subject of research.

If one lets go of the assumptions of materialism, then quantum changes can also be hypothesized as an encounter with the nonmaterial, transpersonal realm of spirit. The clear sense of being in the presence of some holy Other was reported by most of those with epiphanies, but also by 42% of those with insightful quantum changes. (Sometimes, in fact, we found it difficult to classify a story as one or the other. There is a large gray area.) Some named this sacred presence as God, some had other names, and some could give it no name at all. One need not, however, believe in a personal, anthropomorphic God to postulate an encounter with the divine. Within various spiritual traditions, people are believed to have access to a great pool of collective, ancestral wisdom, akin to what Jung called the collective unconscious. Within nondeistic religions such as Buddhism, one experiences a sacred oneness with all of nature. In this way, an encounter with the sacred does not necessarily mean that some divine being took the initiative (although that is how many quantum changers described their experience). It is only that something broke through, whether it be from a personal or collective unconscious, a realm of ancestral wisdom, or a divine being.

What is it that might render us so spiritually receptive at a particular moment? The most common antecedent, as we have seen, was intense pain or emotional distress, a point of desperation or hitting bottom, and that seems to be one important source of receptivity. Yet intense pain does not yield quantum change for most of those who suffer it, so again we must ask why these particular people at this particular time had such an experience. Although their backgrounds often cried out for release, there is a puzzle as to why quantum changes came to these people and not others. It is a question quantum changers ask themselves: "Why me, and not so many others?" Millions face desperation and suffering similar to that described in their stories. Many bear scars of child abuse all their lives. Substance abuse is widespread. Countless people take to their knees in desperate prayer at times of crisis. Relationships fall apart constantly. Why were these particular people transformed by joy while countless others were not?

Besides personal pain, another common theme involves some conscious decision to be open to the spiritual, although few anticipated what would follow that decision. About a third of our participants told us that someone was praying for them at the time of their quantum change or that they were praying themselves—often crying out for help when all other hope was gone. Yet for others like Scrooge there was nothing at all out of the ordinary going on just before it happened.

None of those we talked with would claim that they had possessed any special wisdom or virtue to set them apart as more deserving. To the contrary, like John Newton, the ex-slave and slave trader sea captain who wrote *Amazing Grace*,[47] they are filled with amazement and gratitude for a blessing to which they had no special claim. To regard quantum change as a divine gift is also to raise the disturbing question of why these people (and not others) were gifted.

For those who believe in God, quantum changes pose a theological puzzle in this regard. The mystical type of quantum change, at least, bears the mark of spiritual intervention. These experiences are not, of course, in themselves a proof of the existence of God or of a spiritual realm beyond material existence. For those who believe in

God, however—as most quantum changers do, at least after their experience—the hand of God is a plausible way to understand what happened to them. Although not all of them gave it the name of God, most people with a mystical quantum change felt the presence of a greater and profoundly loving being beyond themselves and took little or no personal credit for what happened to them. If they are correct, then God or some Other does intervene in some cases, and apparently not on the basis of need or merit alone.

One possible resolution to the "Why me?" dilemma is that God did not, in fact, single the person out for a blessing. Don's story in Chapter 11 resembles several others in his sense that the divine is *always* present, *always* seeking us and desiring relationship. The difference, then, may be in being receptive, in being where we can be open to what is already and always there.

The problem is, in many ways, the same one taken up by Rabbi Harold S. Kushner in When Bad Things Happen to Good People.[48] There is no fair and just answer to why certain people are caught in the cross fire, or in the building when it collapses, or on the airliner when it crashes. For believers, Kushner reasons that if God is truly good and loving, then God must somehow be unable (not unwilling) to intervene in all suffering. In the end, Kushner leaves the problem in the realm of mystery beyond our present comprehension.

THE LIMITS OF CATEGORIES

Before moving on, we caution that the five possible sources of quantum change described above are not meant to be mutually exclusive categories. The stories themselves elude neat categorization. We have chosen not to focus on a taxonomic system for classifying stories, but rather on understanding what the stories have to teach us about human nature.

Don's story (Chapter 11) is a classic mystical experience, but also sounds like a maturational milestone. The experience of "A Mirror and Two Roses" (Chapter 7) has many qualities of a breaking point and could also be understood as a particular-person issue of working through impacted grief. The woman who experienced "Awakening" (Chapter 8) had not been in acute crisis, but her story has many indications of a developing deep discrepancy; yet her experience might also be attributed to a particular-person attribute in that she had been practicing meditation for fifteen years. "Something Like a Star" (Chapter 12) has many hallmarks of a sacred encounter but could also be understood as the eruption of a deep discrepancy. Quantum changes don't fit neatly into boxes. Perhaps they are better understood as tapestries that weave together some but not all common threads.

SUPPORTING QUANTUM CHANGE

For believers and nonbelievers alike, it is worthwhile pondering how and why the remarkable changes described in earlier chapters came to these particular people. The answer may be randomness or the inscrutable acts of God, but it may also be more systematic and comprehensible. If so, this puzzle contains clues for understanding a remarkable form of healing and for making it available to others. We hope, in fact, that this is where our work will ultimately lead.

The five models just described do suggest a number of ways in which others might be involved in and supportive of quantum change. We describe these here as *possible influence roles*—*possible* because we do not yet know enough about the involvement of others to make definite recommendations, and *influence roles* because a broad range of others (not only identified healers) may be influential in the process.

It would be both important and challenging to study the impact of possible influence roles on the process and outcome of quantum change. One complication is that it is no simple matter to know when quantum change is about to happen or needs to happen. To influence the process prospectively, one presumably would need to be there (although there are some conceptions of healing that are not dependent upon time and distance[49]). Using the retrospective inquiry approach described in this book, it could be interesting to ask quantum changers to speculate on people who may have had an important influence on the course of their experience. Another possibility is to study processes of influence in current therapeutic, spiritual, and other experiences that are intended to evoke quantum change. Perhaps some healers (such as the gurus described in Chapters 6 and 9) are particularly gifted in facilitating a quantum change. For those of us with more ordinary healing gifts and motivations, how might we support people in quantum change?

Offering Support

One time-tested role for helpers is to be a *companion* on the journey, to stand with and support the person through the change process. This does not assume that one can or should do anything to influence the course of quantum change. The function may be primarily that of reassurance and reflection. We found that even more than a decade later most quantum changers hungered to talk about their experience. Being a good listener, offering accurate empathic reflections, may be quite helpful in consolidating and understanding a quantum change experience. Another important supportive function is *normalization*. Many of those who told us their stories said they were surprised and greatly relieved to learn that others had had similar experiences. Many have been secretive about their experience, talking to no one about it or to only a few trusted others. We hope that one function of this book will be to normalize the experience of quantum change, giving quantum changers encouragement to talk more openly about these life-changing events.

A third supportive function is to foster *hope*.[50] For those in distress, there is the knowledge that amazing change can and does happen. Perhaps the stories offered in this volume will affirm some measure of hope and faith in the capacity of the human spirit to change, even and especially when things look darkest. A fear reported by some early quantum changers is that their newfound identity might dissipate. Although no guarantee can be given to the individual person, the stories here at least assure us that quantum change can and does endure. Some people knew this right away—that they had passed through a one-way door. Others had been less sure. Yet everyone we interviewed (admittedly a self-selected sample) found that the transformation not only endured but continued and grew over time. Similar testimony is found in the Big Book of AA.[51]

Evoking Wisdom

We didn't encounter much need among quantum changers to be told what to do. They seem to have a deep confidence in an inner wisdom that guides them. We share that confidence. A skilled helper can, however, play a useful role by evoking that wisdom. We know no better tools for doing this than the client-centered counseling skills described by Carl R. Rogers and his colleagues.[52] We find that reflective listening (accurate empathy, active listening) in particular helps the person to explore his or her own experience and to progress further along in the journey. The helping process is not one of instilling wisdom but of evoking it from the person's own experience.

Developing Discrepancy

In part, quantum change seems to emerge from inner conflict, from a clashing of "how I am" and "how I want to be or could be." If salient awareness of this discrepancy is part of what triggers quantum change, then there may be ways of heightening or facilitating such awareness. We believe that the discrepancy that matters is one that arises from within. It comes from experiencing inner contradictions, sometimes at the level of deeply held values. The helping task, then, is to facilitate the discovery process, the experiencing of discrepancies *already present* in the person but somehow sealed off or dissociated in a way that inhibits them from triggering change.

Some believe that change results from *making* people see, from confronting them and *forcing* them to see. This intrusive model, of installing one's own wisdom into another, is quite different from what we mean. The discrepancy that counts is not imposed, not inflicted, but experienced. We have had considerable success in helping people to change specific harmful behaviors in this way through a respectful, person-centered approach known as motivational interviewing.[53] In working with problem drinkers, for example, we may first seek to understand what it is they value and hold dear, what they care about, what matters most to them in life. In this context, sometimes a simple gentle question such as "How does your drinking fit in here?" can call forth a person's own discrepancies in a way that evokes change. Behavior changes when one perceives that it is inconsistent or interfering with roles and goals that are more important. We suspect that broader changes may also be facilitated by exploring intrinsic value discrepancies..

Providing Positive Models

There are times when one person who "believed in me" has played a significant role in transformation. That belief, we think, involves a positive vision of what and how a person *could* be. It may not be based on any hard evidence. Don Quixote had a transforming vision of Aldonza, a prostitute, as the worthy lady Dulcinea. There was no factual basis for his delusion. In fact, all evidence was to the contrary. Yet he provided an alternative vision, a possible self that like Pygmalion's sculpture came to life. It is the fanciful fiction of Miguel de Cervantes, to be sure, yet there is truth in such stories that are so enduring in our culture. Realities often begin with dreams, with imagined possibilities. Most fundamental is belief in the person's inherent worth and value.[54]

To see the positive possibilities in each other is a remarkable gift. At life's turning points people need positive possible selves to whom they can turn.

OPEN QUESTIONS

In addition to suggesting some answers, good research usually brings to awareness new questions. Our study of quantum change to date has certainly left us with unanswered questions. Here are a few of them. Most likely by now you have thought of these and others.

Why These People?

After ten years, we still have no satisfactory answer to why quantum change happened to these particular people, and not to others who seem to fit the same observable patterns or characteristics. As discussed earlier, many people hit bottom, suffer profound loss, reach the end of their rope, live in desperation, and even cry out in prayer, yet no quantum change occurs. It is a question that also haunts some quantum changers.

How Does It Happen?

We have offered in this chapter a variety of possibilities for why quantum changes occur. Yet we are left mostly with a sense of mystery. By what possible mechanism could the diverse and yet similar experiences of these stories occur? What really happened in that "Something Like a Star" moment (Chapter 12)? "Whatever out there cared enough" was one person's way of describing the mystery from which quantum change emanated. Does the source of quantum change lie outside the material reality that we understand through our limited physical senses?

Givers

Just as there are particular recipients of quantum change, are there particular people who have a gift of imparting it? Was the guru of "Taking the AA Train" (Chapter 6) someone who regularly triggers quantum change in those whose lives he touches? Certainly traditional accounts of great spiritual leaders contain stories of lives they changed in a moment's encounter. There are also tales of certain therapists, like Anton Mesmer[55] and Milton H. Erickson,[56] who could evoke sweeping changes in their clients through relatively brief encounters. If such givers do exist, what exactly is their gift?

External Triggers

More generally, are there particular kinds of events that are more likely to trigger a quantum change? External events or objects seemed to play a significant role in some of the stories recounted in this book: a profound loss, a fireplace, a broken neck, a mirror, an abortion, and a runaway daughter. Did these externals just happen to be there at the moment quantum change struck, or did they play some role? Were they incidental "last straws" that set the process in motion, or was there something specifically important about them?

Is Personality Really Changed?

Because personality is conceived of as the relatively enduring nature of a person, it is an important question whether quantum change truly alters personality. Before-and-after personality testing in quantum change might be ideal, but it would require knowing which people are about to have one. The real-life stories we collected certainly suggest changes of a magnitude that would constitute alteration of personality, though perhaps not as total as in the story of Scrooge. What is it about a person that is truly different after quantum change?

A CLOSING COMMENT

No one of the explanations offered in this chapter seems to fully account for quantum change. Perhaps they all contain some part of the truth. Perhaps there is something fundamentally flawed in the way we think about human change. Perhaps we do not yet comprehend enough about psychological and spiritual reality to understand why quantum changes occur.[57] What is truly hopeful is that they *do* occur. The richness of these true stories, like the enduring appeal of *A Christmas Carol*, reminds us that even and especially in times of deep darkness there is the possibility of transformation. Whatever the source of such quantum change, humanity is capable of finding profound joy in the midst of crisis and entirely new life in the belly of despair. It comes even to those not seeking it, not even aware of a need or possibility for such deep renewal. It is as though life delights in taking us by surprise, tapping us on the shoulder and reminding us now and again of how very little we really know of all that is possible.

19

MESSAGES TO HUMANKIND

Now there are some things we all know, but we don't
take'm out and look at'm very often. We all know that
something is eternal. And it ain't houses and it ain't
names, and it ain't earth, and it ain't even the stars. . . .
[E]verybody knows in their bones that *something* is
eternal, and that something has to do with human
beings. All the greatest people ever lived have been
telling us that for five thousand years and yet you'd be
surprised how people are always losing hold of it.
—THORNTON WILDER, *Our Town*[58]

At first we had planned to end this book with the preceding chapter, puzzling from a psychological perspective about why
quantum changes occur. As we reviewed the story transcripts for
this purpose, however, another impression began to emerge. These
women and men differed substantially on just about every personal
dimension one could imagine including age, education, occupation,
social class, ethnic background, personality, and religion. Nevertheless they had experiences that were in many ways similar in form
and content. They described their quantum change events through
widely varying imagery, worldviews, and vocabulary, yet we could
not escape the sense that in important ways we were hearing the
same story over and over again. You may have had the same experience in reading their stories.

Perhaps there are some consistent messages here not only for these particular people but for humankind as well. These extraordinary experiences came to people who generally thought of themselves as ordinary and not particularly meriting the gift they received. As we noted earlier, many of them have wondered, "Why me?"

Looking at the quantum change stories from this perspective, they may contain some lessons for us all. One can read *A Christmas Carol* as an entertaining ghost story, a tale of bizarre events in the life of one fictional character. Within the broader context of the author's lifework, however, it is clear that Charles Dickens intended Scrooge's spirits to haunt us as well. That a human being *can* have such an encounter, and be permanently changed by it, is part of the enduring appeal of the tale.

Suppose, then, that we were to listen to these quantum change stories at a deeper level. What if these are not merely fascinating, stranger-than-fiction experiences that came to real people, to be read and then put on the shelf? Imagine, instead, that within them are some common seeds of truth, messages trying to get through to us all that announce themselves almost but not quite at random in the lives of fellow human beings. What are these truth-full seeds? What is it that we might learn from these extraordinary experiences of ordinary people?

KNOWING OF TRUTH

At the broadest level, the stories tell us that we are not prisoners of the past, not locked into the people we have been. Profound change can and does occur in human lives, sometimes quite rapidly.

They also speak clearly of what has been called "another way of knowing," beyond the usual processes of sensation and reasoning. As a society, we tend to operate by certain implicit rules of evidence, analogous to those used in courtroom law. You are allowed to know that which you have experienced directly through the senses. Seeing is believing. Eye witnesses are the most credible, and subjective impressions or secondhand hearsay count for less than what we know by hearing or overhearing. When we are asked how we know something, the socially expected response is to describe the evidence of the senses and the logical processes by which we arrived at our conclusion. Much of the charm of Arthur Conan Doyle's stories was in how Sherlock Holmes knew things that others did not, through his superb powers of observation and deduction.

Quantum changers seldom say they arrived at the experience by their own powers of logic and observation. Rather, it broke upon then like a sneaker wave, while their backs were turned to the sea. It knocked them over. It came upon them with such force and clarity that they immediately knew it for truth. To be sure, there is variability in this, but the immediate recognition of a truth is quite characteristic of quantum changes. At least at the experiential level, it comes not from logical proof or cumulative observations but in a sudden rush of knowing.

Is such knowing trustworthy? That is not a question often asked by quantum changers themselves. Did Scrooge, on Christmas day, brood over whether he should really believe what the spirits had shown him? Hardly, for he was too busy experiencing the joy and freedom of what he now knew with surety to be so.

Unlike English, the Norwegian language has several verbs for knowing that reflect the degree of certitude, or *how* the person knows. One of them (*å synes*) expresses a feeling or perception about something while recognizing that others may well take a different view. To communicate this in English, we might say, with an inflection, "I *think* so," or add a qualifying phrase such as "at least that's what I think." The verb *å tro* communicates more of a personal assurance that something is true, including issues of faith. *Å mene* expresses a stronger factually based opinion or intellectual conviction that something is so, as might arise in a political disagreement. It is a fourth verb for "to know" (*å vite*) that communicates surety, a confidence right down to the bones that something is true. There is no such word in English, really. Even phrases like "I'm sure" or "I'm absolutely certain" do not fully capture it. This kind of knowing, again, may be communicated by inflection: "I just *know*." Perhaps closest to the quantum change kind of knowing is the phrase, "I know it in my heart."[59]

A picture of quantum change knowing is incomplete, however, without a common companion aspect of these experienced truths. It is a somewhat surprising attribute, not one ordinarily associated with convicted certainty. Most quantum changers seem disinclined to convert or convince others. Ardent proselytism is what one might expect when a person has "seen the truth." A few of the people we met had tried at first to persuade others, but even these tended with time to hold their truth gently and quietly. Some just keep it to themselves. Some share it willingly when asked, but even then there tends to be a respectful sense of "take what is useful to you from my experience and leave the rest." They do not need to convince others in order to be convinced themselves. Often it is those newer to a faith who tend to feel most urgently the need for others to profess the same truth, thus reinforcing their own belief. Quantum changers seem to need no such reassurance by agreement. They *know*.

At this level, quantum changes may have some things to teach us about the knowing of truth itself. One is that *there are different ways of knowing truth*. The scientific method, for example, is a useful and valuable tool for discovering truth. It was through careful observation and logic that thinkers like Nicolaus Copernicus and Galileo Galilei came to be convinced of new truths that contradicted shared certainties of their day. To claim that this is the *only* way of knowing, however, is to ignore experience, and bespeaks a dogmatic certainty that does not itself arise from the scientific method of knowing. As mentioned earlier, Carl G. Jung described an intuitive way of knowing that matches well the experiences of quantum changers, where the process is more like making leaps than proceeding step by step. It is an imaginative (not imaginary) process familiar not only to mystics but also to scientists like Albert Einstein. *There are different ways of knowing truth*. Those who have experienced quantum changes know it well, and often their stories reflect their surprise at this discovery.

The companion lesson, then, seems to be that *truth is not to be imposed*. Having experienced a great turning point and what they often describe as the most important truth of their lives, quantum changers nevertheless seem to be, if anything, careful not to impose it on others:

> *I just found a big inner strength, and I feel confident. Now that I have this inner strength, I want to use it to help people, if they need my guidance, because of my experience. I don't want to try to preach to anybody, or tell them, well, "There is a God because this happened to me." I just feel that that's a very personal thing and it comes to you when it's your time. I don't like to preach to people or anything like that, but I do want to be there for them.*

Another woman said this:

> *I really have a deep religious point of view, but I try not to let that spill over too much in relationships, except in just caring about people and trying to see them as who they are. I try to see the best of them, so that I'm not hampered by fences, by negative boundaries. I don't want my religious point of view to frighten or upset other people, because it can be very expansive. I just want to keep growing.*

The reticence does not arise from any sense of possessiveness, from a miserly "keeping it all for myself." The person might keep silent for fear of being misunderstood or censured, but there is something more here. Perhaps it arises from the very knowledge that there are different ways of knowing and from a respect for others' own searches. We met no one among the quantum changers who conveyed the impression that "I know the one and only Truth, and those who disagree with me are wrong." Rather, the silence of quantum changers has a quality of peacefulness and humility.

BEYOND THE SELF

Many quantum changers, like Scrooge, would allow that before their experience, humility had not been among their prominent traits. A common theme in the aftermath of quantum change is a decentering from self, an abrupt move away from an "I-me-my-mine" self-centered view of the world. For those who had a mystical experience in particular, the event was literally humbling. Some felt themselves briefly in the presence of something much greater than themselves. Some experienced themselves as but a small part of a much larger reality, a drop in the ocean. Insightful quantum changes sometimes center on a letting go of personal control or self-importance.

This points to another common message in quantum changes— that *our day-to-day material reality is but a small part of all that is.* A woman who had been agnostic before her experience said with certainty, "After this, I just really sense that something is there. I really do, and I call it God. I'm not particularly religious, but I call it God. There is just something there, something I can feel." Quantum changers tell us that there is much more than what can be perceived through the physical senses. Often, they touched briefly on another dimension of reality that can be called spiritual. It transcends ordinary experience and knowing, and thus can be quite difficult to put into words. The experience is compelling and long remembered, and can take years to integrate.

As is apparent from a number of the stories, quantum changers also clearly recognize the difference between spirituality and religion. Many had had little religious involvement, at least in recent years, prior to their quantum change. Afterward, some were quite involved in a religion and others were not, but nearly all regarded themselves to be deeply spiritual. It was a faith based not on what they had been taught to believe but on their own direct experience.

POSSESSIONS

After quantum change, particularly of the mystical type, few values changed so consistently and profoundly as that placed on material possessions. No one we spoke with had converted to a more self-centered or indulgent "me first" belief system. While very aware of present experiences and pleasures, they no longer gave much priority to *having* things. They could enjoy that which they did have, but acquiring material possessions seemed unimportant, even antithetical to what they truly valued. Among ranked values, the acquisition of wealth often fell from first place to last.

This devaluing of materialism seems related to having directly experienced another reality. If "this is all there is," then anxious acquisition may seem important. Their life-changing glimpse of something much larger suddenly reduced possessions to irrelevance. None of them had renounced all possessions. It was just that they were no longer attached to them, possessed by them. Instead, they had the common sense that each new day and all of life is a gift. Anxiousness or envy for what is not gave way to awareness and gratitude for what is.

THE NATURE OF SPIRITUAL REALITY

Those who touch another kind of reality during a quantum change usually return from it with a clear memory of its nature. They call what they experienced by many different names—unity, God, the Other, or particular figures or symbols from a cultural tradition. Beyond the names, however, there is substantial agreement about the nature of the spiritual reality they encountered.

It was rare for quantum changers to feel afraid in the presence of the Other. Rather, they felt utterly safe. In a few experiences, the first words they heard, or rather experienced, were some form of "Do not be afraid." It was a sense of safety that lingered even many years later: "I have a clear sense that I will be taken care of, that I don't have to be so dramatically concerned with events. The future will take care of itself."

As described in Chapter 10, the almost universal experience of the Other presence or reality encountered in mystical quantum changes was of utter love and of total acceptance, even if the person felt a heightened awareness of past shortcomings. Not everyone conceived the Other as a being, but for those who did understand their experience in this way, the sense was of a profoundly loving and trustworthy Higher Power to whom they could always turn and to whom they are somehow inwardly connected.

Many also felt moved by their experience to acts of compassion and service to others, usually things that would not even have occurred to them to do before their quantum change. Some have volunteered their time to visit prisoners in jails. Others have gone into the streets to feed and care for the homeless. Such acts were rarely from any sense of requirement. Rather, they were the natural result of experiencing, in essence, that *love is what we are and what we are meant to be.* It is our nature. The vision is one that clashes with modern views of humanity as innately self-serving or as a blank slate neither inherently good nor evil. The experience is that we are already and inherently part of—or intimately linked to, or made in the image of, or bearing the seeds of—something named or nameless that is so vast as to defy our imagination and the fundamental nature of which is a love so great that it simply overwhelms our ability to comprehend it:

> *That one experience changed me. "Transformed" me I think would be more the word. I was not, up to that point, what you would call a devotional, religious, spiritual person at all. After that experience I became a different person. I became a more loving, kind, compassionate person. It was like I hit on some part of me that was this*

*good person. I hadn't been a bad person before, but I just hadn't
been aware of the goodness and kindness in me. I never really tried
to explain it. It was very personal. I don't think I ever talked to
anybody about it before this.*

ACCEPTANCE

Linked to this loving nature, quantum change often leaves a deep
sense of compassionate acceptance, both for others and for oneself.
Among those who had a mystical type of quantum change, this was
often part of what they directly experienced in the midst of their
epiphanies. Such acceptance does not deny or overlook shortcomings. Rather its power seems to be in honestly acknowledging and
forgiving them. Forgiveness, in fact, became a central instrumental
value for many who had experienced quantum change:

> *It was just like I could relate to people differently. I had always
> been comfortable with people and had had a great social life, but it
> seemed like I was no longer so critical of other people. I was more
> loving and compassionate and caring, and less critical, less judg-
> mental, less gossipy, that sort of thing. I was more aware of the
> goodness in people, and everywhere I went I met with love. People
> noticed and were relating to me. I attracted more people than I had
> before, because I was more open to them, and I had a much better
> time, too. I made a lot of friends, and when we moved here I made
> a lot of new friends that I still have. That night just changed my
> whole life.*

INTERCONNECTEDNESS

Finally, across quite diverse experiences, a common experience was
that all people are somehow linked, intimately and profoundly. There
were many ways of expressing this realization. Some directly experienced unity with a great Whole of which all humans are a part. Some
were struck by the absence of separation, of boundaries between
themselves and others. For some, this loss of individual identity ex-
tended to the entire universe and eternity, past limits of time and
space. In the words from a story in Chapter 10: "I became aware that

there is so much out there that we weren't aware of. I felt the reality of so many levels of existence, of being able to tap into it." The common experience, however, was that we are not alone, separate, isolated beings. There is a much greater ultimate sense in which we are literally the same, part of some unity. At the end of his life, Morris Schwartz, the subject of Mitch Albom's *Tuesdays with Morrie*,[60] similarly observed:

> If we saw each other as more alike, we might be very eager to join in one big human family in this world, and to care about the family the way we care about our own. But believe me, when you are dying, you see it is true. We all have the same beginning—birth—and we all have the same ending—death. So how different can we be? Invest in the human family.

Yet the unity that quantum changers often perceive is even more than this sense of universally shared human experience. It is different from the thought that "we are all in the same boat," from the image of separate individuals cast together by common interests and circumstances. Neither is it the image of roped-up mountain climbers, each of whose fate depends on that of all the others on the rope. These are worthy philosophical perspectives, but they are different from what quantum changers perceive. The wave that catches them from behind is the direct *experience* of utter unity. To stretch the metaphor, it is not that we are all *in* the same boat but that we *are* the same boat.

SACRED THEMES

Bringing all of these themes together, the messages so deeply implanted in people by these life-changing experiences overlap with what have been central teachings of the world's great spiritual traditions. In this sense there is no new truth for humankind revealed in quantum change. The messages were, to be sure, new for those who experienced these insights and epiphanies—if not in content, at least in the absolute firsthand knowledge of their truth. Often they had heard the words before but had never heard and experienced their meaning. Perhaps, then, quantum changes are periodic reminders to humankind of what we have already known yet have failed to take seriously:

Tomorrow need not be the same as yesterday.

There are different ways of knowing truth, not limited to the physical senses and logic.

Truth is not to be imposed.

Material reality is but a small part of all that is.

Possessions ought not to possess us.

The nature of God (or whatever name may be given to spiritual reality) is a love and acceptance so profound that it over-whelms our ability to comprehend it.

Love is what we are and what we are meant to be.

Shortcomings are to be met with compassion and forgiveness.

All people are intimately and profoundly linked, part of the same whole.

All of life is a gift, and each day a new opportunity.

EPILOGUE

As we completed this book, an old friend reached the end of his days. After a long life of service as a pastor who had touched countless lives, Ken Eaton lay dying, being ministered to by his own pastor. It was the last conversation they would have. "When I speak at your memorial service," his pastor asked, "what do you want me to say to your friends and family?" Ken did not even pause for thought.

"Just tell them this," he said:

> God is real.
> Life is a gift.
> We are here to love.
> This is not all there is.

He, too, knew.

AFTERWORD

Ernest Kurtz

Do human beings change? Can humans be changed? One time-honored way to understand the reality of change is to listen to people's stories. The first great teachers of psychology were bards, playwrights, and other storytellers. The beginnings of modern psychology as well as classical philosophical psychology flourished using the tools of careful observation (especially of oneself) infused by sensitivity to both quantitative and qualitative differences. Understanding oneself and understanding others were seen to be mutually reinforcing. With no need to measure and to manipulate, those practitioners used all of their senses, especially their common sense.

In this book, Bill Miller and Janet C'de Baca take a large step toward the revival of that tradition among psychologists. Rarely do works in the modern social sciences teach their readers to listen. This book does so. Listening, in contrast with hearing, requires careful attention and active effort. Given normal senses, we hear what is present: we can to a large extent choose either to attend to it or to ignore it, but we do hear it. To listen, however, one must focus attention and to some extent surrender oneself to the source of the sound, be it a speaker or an orchestra.

This tradition of storytelling and story-listening values synthesis

over analysis, comprehensiveness over precision. Books such as this
one offer welcome relief from the arid albeit precise fare that too often claims our ever-more-limited reading time. There are no easy
and few clear and distinct findings here, and those for whom their
intellectual bent is analysis rather than synthesis may find this frustrating. But works like this book urge and enable us to *think* more
than they teach us how to *do* anything.

Miller and C'de Baca point out that "description is far from understanding." Perhaps. But they are connected on the same path: one
who wishes to and works at it can always reach the one from the
other. The case is different with understanding and explanation, certainly with the type of "explanation" that in reality explains away,
but also with that which results in attempts to control.

Faced with mystical experience, understanding and explanation
both fall short and, if wise, stand mute. However, firsthand description by those who have had such experience must be attempted, because the experience of the good must be communicated—or at least
witnessed to. This is, in a way, the "price" of mystical experience for,
the mystic's task is, as Alan Watts mischievously suggested, "to eff
the ineffable."

Mystics, when they speak, use imagery that tells stories. Listening to stories is one way of gathering inductive evidence. It is also
a methodology that requires not only patience but faith and humility—a deep conviction that those to whom we listen have something
to teach us and on their own terms. To learn what they teach one
must be willing to "listen thoroughly," not attempting to fit what one
hears into one's own categories but hoping to absorb from the inside
the other's categories so that one might better participate in his or
her experience.

The very ineffability of the mystical experience leads those who
have experienced it to stretch language in ways that benefit us all.
Stories of change employ the imagery of metaphor to wrap the un-
speakable in memorable images. The language of "unburdening," for
example, conveys the sense of an oppressively heavy weight being
lifted. The kinesthetic sense, indeed, often seems the most applica-
ble image, despite the continuance of the ancient popular philosophical metaphors of seeing and knowing. Such happy phrases as "a
feeling of light," with their blending of the tactile and visual senses,
draw us beyond the point, however blurred, of change itself. They
remind those who listen thoroughly to look to context, to see what

follows as well as what preceded. Quantum change, as this book illuminates, is a life-change.

There are many contexts of change, but anyone who has the good fortune to know, or to work with, recovered alcoholics knows the reality that people do change-and the reality that people do *not* change. For change, which is different from complete annihilation and total creation, implies something that remains stable, something in which the change takes place.

Change, then, attests to the "both/and"-ness of the human condition. We are not either-or beings: to be human is to be *both* more and less than "merely human." Heraclitus posited that all things change—*panta hrei*. The ancient Greek's "flow" thus implied both the sameness of a river and the differences of the water moving in it.

And so it goes, and thus it flows. There will always be some people who will meditate on these matters. Or might it be truer to say that there will always be some times when everyone will devote at least a few moments to wondering as well as wandering in this area? Those who do so will find this book stimulating as well as truthful.

AN INVITATION

It has been our experience that as we have talked and written about quantum change, others have come to tell us their stories. We welcome letters describing other experiences of this kind, either anonymously or with contact information to use should we decide to pursue further the study of quantum change. Send stories and correspondence to:

William R. Miller, PhD
Department of Psychology
The University of New Mexico
Albuquerque, NM, USA 87131-1161

Appendix

VALUES: WHAT MATTERS MOST TO YOU?[61]

From the following values, identify your top ten, then place them in order of priority.

ACCEPTANCE	to be accepted as I am
ACCURACY	to be correct in my opinions and actions
ACHIEVEMENT	to accomplish and achieve
ADVENTURE	to have new and exciting experiences
ATTRACTIVENESS	to be physically attractive
AUTHORITY	to be in charge of others
AUTONOMY	to be self-determining and independent
BEAUTY	to appreciate beauty around me
CARING	to take care of others
COMFORT	to have a pleasant, enjoyable life
COMMITMENT	to make a long-lasting and deep commitment to another person
COMPASSION	to feel and show concern for others
COMPLEXITY	to have a life full of variety and change
CONTRIBUTION	to make a contribution that will last after I am gone
COURTESY	to be polite and considerate to others
CREATIVITY	to have new and original ideas
DEPENDABILITY	to be reliable and trustworthy
DUTY	to carry out my duties and responsibilities
ECOLOGY	to live in harmony with and protect the environment
FAITHFULNESS	to be loyal and reliable in relationships
FAME	to be known and recognized

FAMILY	to have a happy, loving family
FLEXIBILITY	to adjust to new or unusual situations easily
FORGIVENESS	to be forgiving of others
FRIENDS	to have close, supportive friends
FUN	to play and have fun
GENEROSITY	to give what I have to others
GENUINENESS	to behave in a manner that is true to who I am
GOD'S WILL	to seek and obey the will of God
GROWTH	to keep changing and growing
HEALTH	to be physically well and healthy
HELPFULNESS	to be helpful to others
HONESTY	to be truthful and genuine
HOPE	to maintain a positive and optimistic outlook
HUMILITY	to be modest and unassuming
HUMOR	to see the humorous side of myself and the world
INDEPENDENCE	to be free from depending on others
INDUSTRY	to work hard and well at my life tasks
INNER PEACE	to experience personal peace
INTIMACY	to share my innermost experience with others
JUSTICE	to promote equal and fair treatment for all
KNOWLEDGE	to learn and possess valuable knowledge
LEISURE	to take time to relax and enjoy
LOGIC	to live rationally and sensibly
LOVED	to be loved by those close to me
LOVING	to give love to others
MASTERY	to be competent in my everyday activities
MODERATION	to avoid excesses and find a middle ground
MONOGAMY	to have one close, loving relationship
ORDERLINESS	to have a life that is well-ordered and organized
PLEASURE	to have experiences that feel good
POPULARITY	to be well liked by many people
POWER	to have control over others
PURPOSE	to have meaning and direction in my life
REALISM	to see and act realistically and practically
RESPONSIBILITY	to make and carry out important decisions
RISK	to take risks and chances
ROMANCE	to have intense, exciting love in my life
SAFETY	to be safe and secure
SELF-ACCEPTANCE	to like myself as I am
SELF-CONTROL	to be self-disciplined and govern my own activities
SELF-ESTEEM	to feel positive about myself
SELF-KNOWLEDGE	to have a deep, honest understanding of myself

SERVICE	to be of service to others
SEXUALITY	to have an active and satisfying sex life
SIMPLICITY	to live life simply, with minimal needs
SPIRITUALITY	to grow spiritually
STABILITY	to have a life that stays fairly consistent
STRENGTH	to be physically strong
TOLERANCE	to accept and respect those different from me
TRADITION	to follow respected patterns of the past
VIRTUE	to live a morally pure and excellent life
WEALTH	to have plenty of money
WORLD PEACE	to work to promote peace in the world

NOTES

1. Quoted in Alcoholics Anonymous (1976). *Alcoholics Anonymous: The story of how many thousands of men and women have recovered from alcoholism* (3rd ed., p. 27). New York: Alcoholics Anonymous World Services.
2. William James (1902). *The varieties of religious experience.* Cambridge, MA: Harvard University Press.
3. Alcoholics Anonymous (1976); see Note 1. See also Ernest Kurtz's (1988) superb history *A.A.: The Story* (a revised edition of his 1979 volume *Not God: A history of Alcoholics Anonymous*). San Francisco: Harper & Row.
4. William James (1902, p. 217); see Note 2.
5. Lewis R. Rambo (1993). *Understanding religious conversion.* New Haven, CT: Yale University Press. See also Ralph W. Hood, Jr., Bernard Spilka, and Richard Gorsuch (1996). *The psychology of religion: An empirical approach* (2nd ed.). New York: Guilford Press.
6. James E. Loder (1981). *The transforming moment: Understanding convictional experiences* (p. 32). New York: Harper & Row.
7. William R. Miller and Janet C'de Baca (1994). Quantum change: Toward a psychology of transformation. In Todd F. Heatherton and Joel L. Weinberger (Eds.), *Can personality change?* (pp. 253–280). Washington, DC: American Psychological Association.
8. Alexander Woodcock and Monte Davis (1978). *Catastrophe theory: A revolutionary new way of understanding how things change* (p. 9). New York: Viking Penguin.

9. Quoted in Ernest Kurtz (1988, p. 20); see Note 3.

10. Abraham H. Maslow (1971). *The farther reaches of human nature* (p. 348). New York: Viking Compass (emphasis in the original).

11. Quoted by Thomas E. Mails (1990) in *Fools Crow* (p. 51). Lincoln: University of Nebraska Press.

12. In fact, excellent research on natural change has been underway for more than two decades. See Mark B. Sobell and Linda C. Sobell (1998). Guiding self-change. In William R. Miller and Nick H. Heather (Eds.), *Treating addictive behaviors* (2nd ed., pp. 189–202). New York: Plenum Press.

13. The centrality of control issues in psychotherapy and change is thoughtfully discussed by Deane H. Shapiro, Jr., and John Astin (1998) in *Control therapy: An integrative approach to psychotherapy, health, and healing.* New York: Wiley.

14. Brenda S. Cole and Kenneth I. Pargament (1999). Spiritual surrender: A paradoxical path to control. In William R. Miller (Ed.), *Integrating spirituality into treatment: Resources for practitioners* (pp. 179–216). Washington, DC: American Psychological Association.

15. Quoted in Ernest Kurtz (1988, pp. 19–20); see Note 3.

16. Alcoholics Anonymous (1976, p. 27); see Note 1.

17. William James (1902); see Note 2.

18. These are compiled in Wayne Oates's 1973 volume *The psychology of religion* (p. 117). Waco, TX: Word Books. The original document is Walter Pahnke (1963). *Drugs and mysticism: An analysis of the relationship between psychedelic drugs and mystical consciousness.* Doctoral dissertation, Harvard University. Pahnke's dissertation was supervised by Timothy Leary. See also Rick Doblin (1991). Pahnke's "Good Friday experiment": A long-term follow-up and methodological critique. *Journal of Transpersonal Psychology, 23,* 1–28.

19. Paul Tillich (1948). You are accepted. In *The shaking of the foundations* (p. 162). New York: Scribner's.

20. Abraham H. Maslow (1968). *Toward a psychology of being* (2nd ed., p. 102). New York: Van Nostrand Reinhard (emphasis in original).

21. Meyer Friedman and Ray H. Rosenman (1974). *Type A behavior and your heart.* New York: Knopf.

22. Abraham H. Maslow (1968, p. 88); see Note 20.

23. Don Eaton can be contacted through Small Change, 1164 NW Weybridge Way, Beaverton, OR, USA 97006.

24. Abraham H. Maslow (1971, p. 53); see Note 10.

25. Abraham H. Maslow (1971, p. 49); see Note 10.

26. This paradox is captured superbly in *The spirituality of imperfection* by Ernest Kurtz and Kathleen Ketcham (1992). New York: Bantam Books.

27. From Carl G. Jung (1953). *The collected works of Carl G. Jung,* Vol. 7,

Two essays on analytical psychology (second essay). Translated by R. F. C. Hull. Princeton, NJ: Bollingen Foundation.

28. Abraham H. Maslow (1968, p. 81); see Note 20.
29. Rick Doblin (1991, p. xx); see Note 18.
30. Yuichiro Miura. (1978). *The man who skied down Everest*. New York: Harper & Row.
31. William James (1902, p. 218) in his lecture on "Conversion"; see Note 2.
32. For example, a sudden transformation of personality and identity was well documented by David H. Barlow, Gene G. Abel, & Edward G. Blanchard (1977). Gender identity change in a transsexual: An exorcism. *Archives of Sexual Behavior, 6*, 387–395.
33. Frederick H. Kanfer (1970). Self-regulation: Research, issues, and speculations. In Charles Neuringer and J. L. Michael (Eds.), *Behavior modification in clinical psychology* (pp. 178–220). New York: Appleton-Century-Crofts. See also Frederick H. Kanfer (1987). Self-regulation and behavior. In H. Heckhausen, P. M. Gollwitzer, and F. E. Weinert (Eds.), *Jenseits des Rubikon* (pp. 286–299). Heidelberg: Springer-Verlag.
34. William R. Miller and Janice M. Brown (1993). Self-regulation as a conceptual basis for the prevention and treatment of addictive behaviours. In Nick H. Heather, William R. Miller, and Janet Greeley (Eds.), *Self-control and the addictive behaviours* (pp. 3–79). Botany, New South Wales, Australia: Maxwell Macmillan.
35. Carl R. Rogers (1959). A theory of therapy, personality, and interpersonal relationships as developed in the client-centered framework. In Sigmund Koch (Ed.), *Psychology: The study of a science: Vol. 3. Formulations of the person and the social context* (pp. 184–256). New York: McGraw-Hill.
36. Roy F. Baumeister (1994). The crystallization of discontent in the process of major life change. In Todd F. Heatherton & Joel L. Weinberger (Eds.), *Can personality change?* (pp. 281–297). Washington, DC: American Psychological Association; quotation from p. 282.
37. Milton Rokeach (1973). *The nature of human values*. New York: Free Press.
38. Among others, Roberto Assagioli (1971), the progenitor of *Psychosynthesis* (New York: Penguin Books), faulted psychodynamic theorists for exploring only the lower cellar of the house (the unconscious) and not the attic, the higher forms of consciousness to which people have access.
39. Lawrence Kohlberg (1984). *The psychology of moral development: The nature and validity of moral stages*. San Francisco: Harper & Row.
40. James W. Fowler (1981). *Stages of faith: The psychology of human development and the quest for meaning*. San Francisco: Harper & Row.

41. Abraham H. Maslow (1968, p. 79); see Note 20.

42. Abraham H. Maslow (1968, p. 97); see Note 20.

43. P. V. Robb (1982). Conversion as a human experience. *Studies in the Spirituality of Jesuits, 14*(3), 1–50.

44. William James (1902, p. 265); see Note 2.

45. Isabel B. Myers and Mary H. McCaulley (1985). *Manual: A guide to the development and use of the Myers–Briggs Type Indicator.* Palo Alto, CA: Consulting Psychologists Press.

46. Others have argued that psychosis similarly is an important experience that one should at least be allowed the choice of having. R. D. Laing has particularly been a strong voice in this regard.

47. See Brian H. Edwards (1975). *Through many dangers.* Welwyn, Hertfordshire, UK: Evangelical Press.

48. Rabbi Harold S. Kushner (1989). *When bad things happen to good people.* New York: Schocken Books.

49. Larry Dossey (1993). *Healing words: The power of prayer and the practice of medicine.* San Francisco: Harper.

50. Carolina E. Yahne and William R. Miller (1999). Evoking hope. In William R. Miller (Ed.), *Integrating spirituality into treatment: Resources for practitioners* (pp. 217–233). Washington, DC: American Psychological Association.

51. See Note 1.

52. Charles B. Truax and Robert R. Carkhuff (1967). *Toward effective counseling and psychotherapy.* Chicago: Aldine. See also Thomas Gordon and W. Sterling Edwards (1995). *Making the patient your partner.* Westport, CT: Auburn House. And J. T. Hart and T. M. Tomlinson (Eds.). (1970). *New directions in client-centered therapy.* Boston: Houghton Mifflin.

53. William R. Miller and Stephen Rollnick (1991). *Motivational interviewing: Preparing people to change addictive behavior.* New York: Guilford Press. See also Stephen Rollnick and William R. Miller (1995). What is motivational interviewing? *Behavioural and Cognitive Psychotherapy, 23*, 325–334.

54. See Carl R. Rogers (1964). Toward a modern approach to values: The valuing process in the mature person. *Journal of Abnormal and Social Psychology, 68*, 160–167.

55. On Mesmer, see Benjamin Franklin (1784). *Report of Dr. Benjamin Franklin, and other commissioners, charged by the King of France, with the examination of animal magnetism, as now practised in Paris.* London: Johnson.

56. Milton H. Erickson, John Grinder, Judith Delozier, and Richard Bandler (1997). *Patterns of the hypnotic techniques of Milton H. Erickson, M.D.* (Vol. 2). Portland, OR: Metamorphosis Press.

57. Nearly a century ago, William James struggled with the same parting of the ways between psychological and theological viewpoints when *describing* transformational change gives way to *explaining* it: "Psychology and religion are thus in perfect harmony up to this point, since both admit that there are forces seemingly outside of the conscious individual that bring redemption to his life. Nevertheless psychology, defining these forces as 'subconscious' and speaking of their effects, as due to 'incubation,' or 'cerebration,' implies that they do not transcend the individual's personality; and herein she diverges from Christian theology, which insists that they are direct supernatural operations of the Deity. I propose to you that we do not yet consider this divergence final, but leave the question for a while in abeyance—continued inquiry may enable us to get rid of some of the apparent discord" (1902, p. 234); see Note 2.

58. Thornton Wilder (1938). *Our town: A play in three acts* (p. 81). New York: Harper & Row.

59. Special thanks to Tom Barth for helping to clarify the shades of meaning that distinguish these Norwegian verbs.

60. Mitch Albom (1997). *Tuesdays with Morrie* (pp. 156–157). New York: Doubleday.

61. Besides being longer, this list differs somewhat in content from the list used in the quantum change study. We gratefully acknowledge the assistance of Dr. Daniel B. Matthews in clarifying and expanding our original list.

INDEX

ABOUT THE AUTHORS

William R. Miller, PhD, is Emeritus Distinguished Professor of Psychology and Psychiatry at the University of New Mexico. He has published 40 books, including *Motivational Interviewing*, and his many scientific publications reflect his interests in the psychology of change, the treatment of addictions, and the interface of psychology and spirituality. The Institute for Scientific Information lists him as one of the world's most cited scientists.

Janet C'de Baca, PhD, is a 1999 graduate of the doctoral program in clinical psychology at the University of New Mexico. That year she began a career as a research scientist with the Behavioral Health Research Center of the Southwest. Her areas of scientific interest include addictive behaviors, youth assessment and behavioral interventions, and cross-cultural issues.